A Wanderer in Florence

E. V. (Edward Verrall) Lucas

Curated Edition

Edited by David Nguyen

Edited by David Nguyen.

Contents

Synopsis

"A Wanderer in Florence" by E. V. Lucas is a travelogue that was likely written in the early 20th century. The narrative engages with the rich artistic and historical heritage of Florence, focusing particularly on the Duomo, its construction, and the prominent figures connected to it. It introduces readers to the enchanting qualities of Florence, shaped by the Renaissance's greatest minds, and hints at various architectural marvels that define the cityscape. The opening of the book begins with a preface that expresses the author's intention to convey the beauty and significance of Florence through its artistic achievements and the warmth of its people. Lucas emphasizes the Duomo, or Cathedral of S. Maria del Fiore, describing its grandeur and contrasting its exterior ornamentation with the hushed sanctity of its interior. The first chapter delves into the history of the Duomo, detailing its construction under notable architects like Arnolfo di Cambio and Giotto, while also highlighting the artistic legacy of figures like Brunelleschi and Donatello. This setup not only transports readers to the heart of Florence but also ignites curiosity about the cultural narratives intertwined with its landmarks.

CHAPTER I

THE Duomo I: Its Construction

The City of the Miracle–The Marble Companions–Twilight and Immensity–Arnolfo di Cambio–Dante's seat–Ruskin's "Shepherd"–Giotto the various–Giotto's fun–The indomitable Brunelleschi–Makers of Florence–The present façade.

All visitors to Florence make first for the Duomo. Let us do the same.

The real name of the Duomo is the Cathedral of S. Maria del Fiore, or St. Mary of the Flowers, the flower being the Florentine lily. Florence herself is called the City of Flowers, and that, in the spring and summer, is a happy enough description. But in the winter it fails. A name appropriate to all the seasons would be the City of the Miracle, the miracle being the Renaissance. For though all over Italy traces of the miracle are apparent, Florence was its very home and still can point to the greatest number of its achievements. Giotto (at the beginning of this quickening movement) may at Assisi have been more inspired as a painter; but here is his campanile and here are his S. Maria Novella and S. Croce frescoes. Fra Angelico and Donatello (in the midst of it) were never more inspired than here, where they worked and died. Michelangelo (at the end of it) may be more surprising in the Vatican; but here are his wonderful Medici tombs. How it came about that between the years 1300 and 1500 Italian soil–and chiefly Tuscan soil–threw up such masters, not only with the will and spirit to do what they did but with the power too, no one will ever be able to explain. But there it is. In the history of the world two centuries were suddenly given mysteriously to the activities of Italian men of humane genius and as suddenly the Divine gift was withdrawn. And to see the very flower of these two centuries it is to Florence we must go.

It is best to enter the Piazza del Duomo from the Via de' Martelli, the Via de' Cerretani, the Via Calzaioli, or the Via Pecori, because then one comes instantly upon the campanile too. The upper windows–so very lovely–may have been visible at the end of the streets, with Brunelleschi's warm dome high in the sky beside them, but that was not to diminish the effect of the first sight of the whole. Duomo and campanile make as fair a couple as ever builders brought together: the immense comfortable church so solidly set upon the earth, and at its side this delicate, slender marble creature, all gaiety and lightness, which as surely springs from roots within the earth. For one cannot be long in Florence, looking at this tower every day and many times a day, both from near and far, without being perfectly certain that it grows–and from a bulb, I think–and was never really built at all, whatever the records may aver.

The interior of the Duomo is so unexpected that one has the feeling of having entered, by some extraordinary chance, the wrong building. Outside it was so garish with its coloured marbles, under the southern sky; outside, too, one's ears were filled with all the shattering noises in which Florence is an adept; and then, one step, and behold nothing but vast and silent gloom. This surprise is the more emphatic if one happens already to have been in the Baptistery. For the Baptistery is also coloured marble without, yet within it is coloured marble and mosaic too: there is no disparity; whereas in the Duomo the walls have a Northern grey and the columns are brown. Austerity and immensity join forces.

When all is said the chief merit of the Duomo is this immensity. Such works of art as it has are not very noticeable, or at any rate do not insist upon being seen; but in its vastness it overpowers. Great as are some of the churches of Florence, I suppose three or four of them could be packed within this one. And mere size with a dim light and a savour of incense is enough: it carries religion. No need for masses and chants or any ceremony whatever: the world is shut out, one is on terms with the infinite. A forest exercises the same spell; among mountains one feels it; but in such a cathedral as the Duomo one feels it perhaps most of all, for it is the work of man, yet touched with mystery and wonder, and the knowledge that man is the author of such a marvel adds to its greatness.

The interior is so dim and strange as to be for a time sheer terra incognita, and to see a bat flitting from side to side, as I have often done even in the morning, is to receive no shock. In such a twilight land there must naturally be bats, one thinks. The darkness is due not to lack of windows but to time. The windows are there, but they have become opaque. None of the coloured ones in the aisle allows more than a filtration of light through it; there are only the plain, circular ones high up and those rich, coloured, circular ones under the dome to do the work. In a little while, however, one's eyes not only become accustomed to the twilight but are very grateful for it; and beginning to look inquiringly about, as they ever do in this city of beauty, they observe, just inside, an instant reminder of the antiseptic qualities of Italy. For by the first great pillar stands a receptacle for holy water, with a pretty and charming angelic figure upon it, which from its air of newness you would think was a recent gift to the cathedral by a grateful Florentine. It is six hundred years old and perhaps was designed by Giotto himself.

The emptiness of the Duomo is another of its charms. Nothing is allowed to impair the vista as you stand by the western entrance: the floor has no chairs; the great columns rise from it in the gloom as if they, too, were rooted. The walls, too, are bare, save for a few tablets.

The history of the building is briefly this. The first cathedral of Florence was the Baptistery, and S. John the Baptist is still the patron saint of the city. Then in 1182 the cathedral was transferred to S. Reparata, which stood on part of the site of the Duomo, and in 1294 the decision to rebuild S. Reparata magnificently was arrived at, and Arnolfo di Cambio was instructed to draw up plans. Arnolfo, whom we see not only on a tablet in the left aisle, in relief, with his plan, but also more than life size, seated beside Brunelleschi on the Palazzo de' Canonici on the south side of the cathedral, facing the door, was then sixty-two and an architect of great reputation. Born in 1232, he had studied under Niccolo Pisano, the sculptor of the famous pulpit at Pisa (now in the museum there), of that in the cathedral in Siena, and of the fountain at Perugia (in all of which Arnolfo probably helped), and the designer of many buildings all over Italy. Arnolfo's own unaided sculpture may be seen at its best in the ciborium in S. Paolo Fuori le Mura in Rome; but it is chiefly as an architect that he is now known. He had already given Florence her extended walls and some of her most beautiful buildings–the Or San Michele and the Badia–and simultaneously he designed S. Croce and the Palazzo Vecchio. Vasari has it that Arnolfo was assisted on the Duomo by Cimabue; but that is doubtful.

The foundations were consecrated in 1296 and the first stone laid on September 8th, 1298, and no one was more interested in its early progress than a young, grave lawyer who used to sit on a stone seat on the south side and watch the builders, little thinking how soon he was to be driven from Florence for ever. This seat–the Sasso di Dante–was still to be seen when Wordsworth visited Florence in 1837, for he wrote a sonnet in which he tells us that he in reverence sate there too, "and, for a moment, filled that empty Throne". But one can do so no longer, for the place which it occupied has been built over and only a slab in the wall with an inscription (on the house next the Palazzo de' Canonici) marks the site.

Arnolfo died in 1310, and thereupon there seems to have been a cessation or slackening of work, due no doubt to the disturbed state of the city, which was in the throes of costly wars and embroilments. Not until 1332 is there definite news of its progress, by which time the work had passed into the control of the Arte della Lana; but in that year, although Florentine affairs were by no means as flourishing as they should be, and a flood in the Arno had just destroyed three or four of the bridges, a new architect was appointed, in the person of the most various and creative man in the history of the Renaissance–none other than Giotto himself, who had already received the commission to design the campanile which should stand at the cathedral's side.

Giotto was the son of a small farmer at Vespignano, near Florence. He was instructed in art by Cimabue, who discovered him drawing a lamb on a stone while herding sheep, and took him as his pupil. Cimabue, of whom more is said, together with more of Giotto as a painter, in the chapter on the Accademia, had died in 1302, leaving Giotto far beyond all living artists, and Giotto, between the age of fifty and sixty, was now residing in Cimabue's house. He had already painted frescoes in the Bargello (introducing his friend Dante), in S. Maria Novella, S. Croce, and elsewhere in Italy, particularly in the upper and lower churches at Assisi, and at the Madonna dell' Arena chapel at Padua when Dante was staying there during his exile. In those days no man was painter only or architect only; an all-round knowledge of both arts and crafts was desired by every ambitious youth who was attracted by the wish to make beautiful things, and Giotto was a universal master. It was not then surprising that on his settling finally in Florence he should be invited to design a campanile to stand for ever beside the cathedral, or that he should be appointed superintendent of the cathedral works.

Giotto did not live to see even his tower completed–it is the unhappy destiny of architects to die too soon–but he was able during the four years left him to find time for certain accessory decorations, of which more will be said later, and also to paint for S. Trinità the picture which we shall see in the Accademia, together with a few other works, since perished, for the Badia and S. Giorgio. He died in 1336 and was buried in the cathedral, as the tablet, with Benedetto da Maiano's bust of him, tells. He is also to be seen full length, in stone, in a niche at the Uffizi; but the figure is misleading, for if Vasari is to be trusted (and for my part I find it amusing to trust him as much as possible) the master was insignificant in size.

Giotto has suffered, I think, in reputation, from Ruskin, who took him peculiarly under his wing, persistently called him "the Shepherd," and made him appear as something between a Sunday-school superintendent and the Creator. The "Mornings in Florence" and "Giotto and his Works in Padua" so insist upon the artist's holiness and conscious purpose in all he did that his genial worldliness, shrewdness, and humour, as brought out by Dante, Vasari, Sacchetti, and Boccaccio, are utterly excluded. What we see is an intense saint where really was a very robust man. Sacchetti's story of Giotto one day stumbling over a pig that ran between his legs and remarking, "And serve me right; for I've made thousands with the help of pigs' bristles and never once given them even a cup of broth," helps to adjust the balance; while to his friend Dante he made a reply, so witty that the poet could not forget his admiration, in answer to his question how was it that Giotto's pictures were so beautiful and his six children so ugly; but I must leave the reader to hunt it for himself, as these are modest pages. Better still, for its dry humour, was his answer to King Robert of Naples, who had commanded him to that city to paint some Scriptural scenes, and, visiting the artist while he worked, on a very hot day, remarked, "Giotto, if I were you I should leave off painting for a while". "Yes," replied Giotto, "if I were you I should."

To Giotto happily we come again and again in this book. Enough at present to say that upon his death in 1336 he was buried, like Arnolfo, in the cathedral, where the tablet to his memory may be studied, and was succeeded as architect, both of the church and the tower, by his friend and assistant, Andrea Pisano, whose chief title to fame is his Baptistery doors and the carving, which we are soon to examine, of the scenes round the base of the campanile. He, too, died–in 1348–before the tower was finished.

Francesco Talenti was next called in, again to superintend both buildings, and not only to superintend but to extend the plans of the cathedral. Arnolfo and Giotto had both worked upon a smaller scale; Talenti determined the present floor dimensions. The revised façade was the work of a committee of artists, among them Giotto's godson and disciple, Taddeo Gaddi, then busy with the Ponte Vecchio, and Andrea Orcagna, whose tabernacle we shall see at Or San Michele. And so the work went on until the main structure was complete in the thirteen-seventies.

Another longish interval then came, in which nothing of note in the construction occurred, and the next interesting date is 1418, when a competition for the design for the dome was announced, the work to be given eventually to one Filippo Brunelleschi, then an ambitious and nervously determined man, well known in Florence as an architect, of forty-one. Brunelleschi, who, again according to Vasari, was small, and therefore as different as may be from the figure which is seated on the clergy house opposite the south door of the cathedral, watching his handiwork, was born in 1377, the son of a well-to-do Florentine of good family who wished to make him a notary. The boy, however, wanted to be an artist, and was therefore placed with a goldsmith, which was in those days the natural course. As a youth he attempted everything, being of a pertinacious and inquiring mind, and he was also a great debater and student of Dante; and, taking to sculpture, he was one of those who, as we shall see in a later chapter, competed for the commission for the Baptistery gates. It was indeed his failure in that competition which decided him to concentrate on architecture. That he was a fine sculptor his competitive design, now preserved in the Bargello, and his Christ crucified in S. Maria Novella, prove; but in leading him to architecture the stars undoubtedly did rightly.

It was in 1403 that the decision giving Ghiberti the Baptistery commission was made, when Brunelleschi was twenty-six and Donatello, destined to be his life-long friend, was seventeen; and when Brunelleschi decided to go to Rome for the study of his new branch of industry, architecture, Donatello went too. There they worked together, copying and measuring everything of beauty, Brunelleschi having always before his mind the problem of how to place a dome upon the cathedral of his native city. But, having a shrewd knowledge of human nature and immense patience, he did not hasten to urge upon the authorities his claims as the heaven-born architect, but contented himself with smaller works, and even assisted his rival Ghiberti with his gates, joining at that task Donatello and Luca della Robbia, and giving lessons in perspective to a youth who was to do more than any man after Giotto to assure the great days of painting and become the exemplar of the finest masters–Masaccio.

It was not until 1419 that Brunelleschi's persistence and belief in his own powers satisfied the controllers of the cathedral works that he might perhaps be as good as his word and was the right man to build the dome; but at last he was able to begin. [1] For the story of his difficulties, told minutely and probably with sufficient accuracy, one must go to Vasari: it is well worth reading, and is a lurid commentary on the suspicions and jealousies of the world. The building of the dome, without scaffolding, occupied fourteen years, Brunelleschi's device embracing two domes, one within the other, tied together with stone for material support and strength. It is because of this inner dome that the impression of its size, from within the cathedral, can disappoint. Meanwhile, in spite of all the wear and tear of the work, the satisfying of incredulous busy bodies, and the removal of such an incubus as Ghiberti, who because he was a superb modeller of bronze reliefs was made for a while joint architect with a salary that Brunelleschi felt should either be his own or no one's, the little man found time also to build beautiful churches and cloisters all over Florence. He lived to see his dome finished and the cathedral consecrated by Pope Eugenius IV in 1436, dying ten years later. He was buried in the cathedral, and his adopted son and pupil, Buggiano, made the head of him on the tablet to his memory.

Brunelleschi's lantern, the model of which from his own hand we shall see in the museum of the cathedral, was not placed on the dome until 1462. The copper ball above it was the work of Verrocchio. In 1912 there are still wanting many yards of stone border to the dome.

Of the man himself we know little, except that he was of iron tenacity and lived for his work. Vasari calls him witty, but gives a not good example of his wit; he seems to have been philanthropic and a patron of poor artists, and he grieved deeply at the untimely death of Masaccio, who painted him in one of the Carmine frescoes, together with Donatello and other Florentines.

As one walks about Florence, visiting this church and that, and peering into cool cloisters, one's mind is always intent upon the sculpture or paintings that may be preserved there for the delectation of the eye. The tendency is to think little of the architect who made the buildings where they are treasured. Asked to name the greatest makers of this beautiful Florence, the ordinary visitor would say Michelangelo, Giotto, Raphael, Donatello, the della Robbias, Ghirlandaio, and Andrea del Sarto: all before Brunelleschi, even if he named him at all. But this is wrong. Not even Michelangelo did so much for Florence as he. Michelangelo was no doubt the greatest individualist in the whole history of art, and everything that he did grips the memory in a vice; but Florence without Michelangelo would still be very nearly Florence, whereas Florence without Brunelleschi is unthinkable. No dome to the cathedral, first of all; no S. Lorenzo church or cloisters; no S. Croce cloisters or Pazzi chapel; no Badia of Fiesole. Honour where honour is due. We should be singing the praises of Filippo Brunelleschi in every quarter of the city.

After Brunelleschi the chief architect of the cathedral was Giuliano da Maiano, the artist of the beautiful intarsia woodwork in the sacristy, and the uncle of Benedetto da Maiano who made the S. Croce pulpit.

The present façade is the work of the architect Emilio de Fabris, whose tablet is to be seen on the left wall. It was finished in 1887, five hundred and more years after the abandonment of Arnolfo's original design and three hundred and more years after the destruction of the second one, begun in 1357 and demolished in 1587. Of Arnolfo's façade the primitive seated statue of Boniface VIII (or John XXII) just inside the cathedral is, with a bishop in one of the sacristies, the only remnant; while of the second façade, for which Donatello and other early Renaissance sculptors worked, the giant S. John the Evangelist, in the left aisle, is perhaps the most important relic. Other statues in the cathedral were also there, while the central figure–the Madonna with enamel eyes–may be seen in the cathedral museum. Although not great, the group of the Madonna and Child now over the central door of the Duomo has much charm and benignancy.

The present façade, although attractive as a mass of light, is not really good. Its patterns are trivial, its paintings and statues commonplace; and I personally have the feeling that it would have been more fitting had Giotto's marble been supplied rather with a contrast than an imitation. As it is, it is not till Giotto's tower soars above the façade that one can rightly (from the front) appreciate its roseate delicacy, so strong is this rival.

CHAPTER II

THE Duomo II: Its Associations

Dante's picture–Sir John Hawkwood–Ancestor and Descendant–The Pazzi Conspiracy–Squeamish Montesecco–Giuliano de' Medici dies–Lorenzo's escape–Vengeance on the Pazzi–Botticelli's cartoon–High Mass–Luca della Robbia–Michelangelo nearing the end–The Miracles of Zenobius–East and West meet in splendour–Marsilio Ficino and the New Learning–Beautiful glass.

Of the four men most concerned in the structure of the Duomo I have already spoken. There are other men held in memory there, and certain paintings and statues, of which I wish to speak now.

The picture of Dante in the left aisle was painted by command of the Republic in 1465, one hundred and sixty-three years after his banishment from the city. Lectures on Dante were frequently delivered in the churches of Florence during the fourteenth and fifteenth centuries, and it was interesting for those attending them to have a portrait on the wall. This picture was painted by Domenico di Michelino, the portrait of Dante being prepared for him by Alessio Baldovinetti, who probably took it from Giotto's fresco in the chapel of the Podestá at the Bargello. In this picture Dante stands between the Inferno and a concentrated Florence in which portions of the Duomo, the Signoria, the Badia, the Bargello, and Or San Michele are visible. Behind him is Paradise. In his hand is the "Divine Comedy". I say no more of the poet here, because a large part of the chapter on the Badia is given to him.

Near the Dante picture in the left aisle are two Donatellos–the massive S. John the Evangelist, seated, who might have given ideas to Michelangelo for his Moses a century and more later; and, nearer the door, between the tablets to De Fabris and Squarciaparello, the so-called Poggio Bracciolini, a witty Italian statesman and Humanist and friend of the Medici, who, however, since he was much younger than this figure at the time of its exhibition, and is not known to have visited Florence till later, probably did not sit for it. But it is a powerful and very natural work, although its author never intended it to stand on any floor, even of so dim a cathedral as this. The S. John, I may say, was brought from the old façade–not Arnolfo's, but the committee's façade–where it had a niche about ten feet from the ground. The Poggio was also on this façade, but higher. It was Poggio's son, Jacopo, who took part in the Pazzi Conspiracy, of which we are about to read, and was very properly hanged for it.

Of the two pictures on the entrance wall, so high as to be imperfectly seen, that on the right as you face it has peculiar interest to English visitors, for (painted by Paolo Uccello, whose great battle piece enriches our National Gallery) it represents Sir John Hawkwood, an English free-lance and head of the famous White Company, who after some successful raids on Papal territory in Provence, put his sword, his military genius, and his bravoes at the service of the highest bidder among the warlike cities and provinces of Italy, and, eventually passing wholly into the employment of Florence (after harrying her for other pay-masters for some years), delivered her very signally from her enemies in 1392. Hawkwood was an Essex man, the son of a tanner at Hinckford, and was born there early in the fourteenth century. He seems to have reached France as an archer under Edward III, and to have remained a free-booter, passing on to Italy, about 1362, to engage joyously in as much fighting as any English commander can ever have had, for some thirty years, with very good pay for it. Although, by all accounts, a very Salomon Brazen-head, Hawkwood had enough dignity to be appointed English Ambassador to Rome, and later to Florence, which he made his home, and where he died in 1394. He was buried in the Duomo, on the north side of the choir, and was to have reposed beneath a sumptuous monument made under his own instructions, with frescoes by Taddeo Gaddi and Giuliano d'Arrigo; but something intervened, and Uccello's fresco was used instead, and this, some sixty years ago, was transferred to canvas and moved to the position in which it now is seen.

Hawkwood's life, briskly told by a full-blooded hand, would make a fine book. One pleasant story at least is related of him, that on being beset by some begging friars who prefaced their mendicancy with the words, "God give you peace," he answered, "God take away your alms"; and, on their protesting, reminded them that such peace was the last thing he required, since should their pious wish come true he would die of hunger. One of the daughters of this fire-eater married John Shelley, and thus became an ancestress of Shelley the poet, who, as it chances, also found a home for a while in this city, almost within hailing distance of his ancestor's tomb and portrait, and here wrote not only his "Ode to the West Wind," but his caustic satire, "Peter Bell the Third".

Hawkwood's name is steeped sufficiently in carnage; but we get to the scene of bloodshed in reality as we approach the choir, for it was here that Giuliano de' Medici was assassinated, as he attended High Mass, on April 26th, 1478, with the connivance, if not actually at the instigation, of Christ's Vicar himself, Pope Sixtus IV. Florentine history is so eventful and so tortuous that beyond the bare outline given in chapter V, I shall make in these pages but little effort to follow it, assuming a certain amount of knowledge on the part of the reader; but it must be stated here that periodical revolts against the power and prestige of the Medici often occurred, and none was more desperate than that of the Pazzi family in 1478, acting with the support of the Pope behind all and with the co-operation of Girolamo Riario, nephew of the Pope, and Salviati, Archbishop of Pisa. The Pazzi, who were not only opposed to the temporal power of the Medici, but were their rivals in business–both families being bankers–wished to rid Florence of Lorenzo and Giuliano in order to be greater both civically and financially. Girolamo wished the removal of Lorenzo and Giuliano in order that hostility to his plans for adding Forli and Faenza to the territory of Imola, which the Pope had successfully won for him against Lorenzo's opposition, might disappear. The Pope had various political reasons for wishing Lorenzo's and Giuliano's death and bringing Florence, always headstrong and dangerous, to heel. While as for Salviati, it was sufficient that he was Archbishop of Pisa, Florence's ancient rival and foe; but he was a thoroughly bad lot anyway. Assassination also was in the air, for Galeazzo Maria Sforza of Milan had been stabbed in church in 1476, thus to some extent paving the way for this murder, since Lorenzo and Sforza, when acting together, had been practically unassailable.

In 1478 Lorenzo was twenty-nine, Giuliano twenty-five. Lorenzo had been at the head of Florentine affairs for nine years and he was steadily growing in strength and popularity. Hence it was now or never.

The conspirators' first idea was to kill the brothers at a banquet which Lorenzo was to give to the great-nephew of the Pope, the youthful Cardinal Raffaello Riario, who promised to be an amenable catspaw. Giuliano, however, having hurt his leg, was not well enough to be present, but as he would attend High Mass, the conspirators decided to act then. That is to say, it was then, in the cathedral, that the death of the Medici brothers was to be effected; meanwhile another detachment of conspirators under Salviati was to rise simultaneously to capture the Signoria, while the armed men of the party who were outside and inside the walls would begin their attacks on the populace. Thus, at the same moment Medici and city would fall. Such was the plan.

The actual assassins were Francesco de' Pazzi and Bernardo Bandini, who were nominally friends of the Medici (Francesco's brother Guglielmo having married Bianca de' Medici, Lorenzo's sister), and two priests named Maffeo da Volterra and Stefano da Bagnone. A professional bravo named Montesecco was to have killed Lorenzo, but refused on learning that the scene of the murder was to be a church. At that, he said, he drew the line: murder anywhere else he could perform cheerfully, but in a sacred building it was too much to ask. He therefore did nothing, but, subsequently confessing, made the guilt of all his associates doubly certain.

When High Mass began it was found that Giuliano was not present, and Francesco de' Pazzi and Bandini were sent to persuade him to come–a Judas-like errand indeed. On the way back, it is said, one of them affectionately placed his arm round Giuliano–to see if he wore a shirt of mail–remarking, to cover the action, that he was getting fat. On his arrival, Giuliano took his place at the north side of the circular choir, near the door which leads to the Via de' Servi, while Lorenzo stood at the opposite side. At the given signal Bandini and Pazzi were to stab Giuliano and the two priests were to stab Lorenzo. The signal was the breaking of the Eucharistic wafer, and at this solemn moment Giuliano was instantly killed, with one stab in the heart and nineteen elsewhere, Francesco so overdoing his attack that he severely wounded himself too; but Lorenzo was in time to see the beginning of the assault, and, making a movement to escape, he prevented the priest from doing aught but inflict a gash in his neck, and, springing away, dashed behind the altar to the old sacristy, where certain of his friends who followed him banged the heavy bronze doors on the pursuing foe. Those in the cathedral, mean-while, were in a state of hysterical alarm; the youthful cardinal was hurried into the new sacristy; Guglielmo de' Pazzi bellowed forth his innocence in loud tones; and his murderous brother and Bandini got off.

Order being restored, Lorenzo was led by a strong bodyguard to the Palazzo Medici, where he appeared at a window to convince the momentarily increasing crowd that he was still living. Meanwhile things were going not much more satisfactorily for the Pazzi at the Palazzo Vecchio, where, according to the plan, the gonfalonier, Cesare Petrucci, was to be either killed or secured. The Archbishop Salviati, who was to effect this, managed his interview so clumsily that Petrucci suspected something, those being suspicious times, and, instead of submitting to capture, himself turned the key on his visitors. The Pazzi faction in the city, meanwhile, hoping that all had gone well in the Palazzo Vecchio, as well as in the cathedral (as they thought), were running through the streets calling "Viva la Libertà!" to be met with counter cries of "Palle! palle!"–the palle being the balls on the Medici escutcheon, still to be seen all over Florence and its vicinity and on every curtain in the Uffizi.

The truth gradually spreading, the city then rose for the Medici and justice began to be done. The Archbishop was handed at once, just as he was, from a window of the Palazzo Vecchio. Francesco de' Pazzi, who had got home to bed, was dragged to the Palazzo and hanged too. The mob meanwhile were not idle, and most of the Pazzi were accounted for, together with many followers–although Lorenzo publicly implored them to be merciful. Poliziano, the scholar-poet and friend of Lorenzo, has left a vivid account of the day. With his own eyes he saw the hanging Salviati, in his last throes, bite the hanging Francesco de Pazzi. Old Jacopo succeeded in escaping, but not for long, and a day or so later he too was hanged. Bandini got as far as Constantinople, but was brought back in chains and hanged. The two priests hid in the Benedictine abbey in the city and for a while evaded search, but being found they were torn to pieces by the crowd. Montesecco, having confessed, was beheaded in the courtyard of the Bargello.

The hanging of the chief conspirators was kept in the minds of the short-memoried Florentines by a representation outside the Palazzo Vecchio, by none other than the wistful, spiritual Botticelli; while three effigies, life size, of Lorenzo–one of them with his bandaged neck–were made by Verrocchio in coloured wax and set up in places where prayers might be offered. Commemorative medals which may be seen in the Bargello, were also struck, and the family of Pazzi was banished and its name removed by decree from the city's archives. Poor Giuliano, who was generally beloved for his charm and youthful spirits, was buried at S. Lorenzo in great state.

I have often attended High Mass in this Duomo choir–the theatre of the Pazzi tragedy–but never without thinking of that scene.

Luca della Robbia's doors to the new sacristy, which gave the young cardinal his safety, had been finished only eleven years. Donatello was to have designed them, but his work at Padua was too pressing. The commission was then given to Michelozzo, Donatello's partner, and to Luca della Robbia, but it seems likely that Luca did nearly all. The doors are in very high relief, thus differing absolutely from Donatello's at S. Lorenzo, which are in very low. Luca's work here is sweet and mild rather than strong, and the panels derive their principal charm from the angels, who, in pairs, attend the saints. Above the door was placed, at the time of Lorenzo's escape, the beautiful cantoria, also by Luca, which is now in the museum of the cathedral, while above the door of the old sacristy was Donatello's cantoria. Commonplace new ones now take their place. In the semicircle over each door is a coloured relief by Luca: that over the bronze doors being the "Resurrection," and the other the "Ascension"; and they are interesting not only for their beauty but as being the earliest-known examples in Luca's newly-discovered glazed terra-cotta medium, which was to do so much in the hands of himself, his nephew Andrea, and his followers, to make Florence still lovelier and the legend of the Virgin Mary still sweeter. But of the della Robbias and their exquisite genius I shall say more later, when we come to the Bargello.

As different as would be possible to imagine is the genius of that younger sculptor, the author of the Pietà at the back of the altar, near where we now stand, who, when Luca finished these bronze doors, in 1467, was not yet born–Michelangelo Buonarroti. This group, which is unfinished, is the last the old and weary Titan ever worked at, and it was meant to be part of his own tomb. Vasari, to whose "Lives of the Painters" we shall be indebted, as this book proceeds, for so much good human nature, and who speaks of Michelangelo with peculiar authority, since he was his friend, pupil, and correspondent, tells us that once when he went to see the sculptor in Rome, near the end, he found him at work upon this Pietà, but the sculptor was so dissatisfied with one portion that he let his lantern fall in order that Vasari might not see it, saying: "I am so old that death frequently drags at my mantle to take me, and one day my person will fall like this lantern". The Pietà is still in deep gloom, as the master would have liked, but enough is revealed to prove its pathos and its power.

In the east end of the nave is the chapel of S. Zenobius, containing a bronze reliquary by Ghiberti, with scenes upon it from the life of this saint, so important in Florentine religious history. It is, however, very hard to see, and should be illuminated. Zenobius was born at Florence in the reign of Constantine the Great, when Christianity was by no means the prevailing religion of the city, although the way had been paved by various martyrs. After studying philosophy and preaching with much acceptance, Zenobius was summoned to Rome by Pope Damasus. On the Pope's death he became Bishop of Florence, and did much, says Butler, to "extirpate the kingdom of Satan". The saint lived in the ancient tower which still stands–one of the few survivors of Florence's hundreds of towers–at the corner of the Via Por S. Maria (which leads from the Mercato Nuovo to the Ponte Vecchio) and the Via Lambertesca. It is called the Torre de' Girolami, and on S. Zenobius' day May 25th is decorated with flowers, and since never are so many flowers in the city of flowers as at that time, it is a sight to see. The remains of the saint were moved to the Duomo, although it had not then its dome, from S. Lorenzo, in 1330, and the simple column in the centre of the road opposite Ghiberti's first Baptistery doors was erected to mark the event, since on that very spot, it is said, stood a dead elm tree which, when the bier of the saint chanced to touch it, immediately sprang to life again and burst into leaf; even, the enthusiastic chronicler adds, into flower. The result was that the tree was cut completely to pieces by relic hunters, but the column by the Baptistery, the work of Brunelleschi (erected on the site of an earlier one), fortunately remains as evidence of the miracle. Ghiberti, however, did not choose this miracle but another for representation; for not only did Zenobius dead restore animation, but while he was himself living he resuscitated two boys. The one was a ward of his own; the second was an ordinary Florentine, for whom the same modest boon was craved by his sorrowing parents. It is one of these scenes of resuscitation which Ghiberti has designed in bronze, while Ridolfo Ghirlandaio painted it in a picture in the Uffizi. We shall see S. Zenobius again in the fresco by Ridolfo's father, the great Ghirlandaio, in the Palazzo Vecchio; while the portrait on the first pillar of the left aisle, as one enters the cathedral is of Zenobius too.

The date of the Pazzi Conspiracy was 1478. A few years later the same building witnessed the extraordinary effects of Savonarola's oratory, when such was the terrible picture he drew of the fate of unregenerate sinners that his listeners' hair was said actually to rise with fright. Savonarola came towards the end of the Renaissance, to give it its death-blow. By contrast there is a tablet on the right wall of the cathedral in honour of one who did much to bring about the paganism and sophistication against which the impassioned reformer uttered his fiercest denunciations: Marsilio Ficino (1433-1491), the neo-Platonist protegé of Cosimo de' Medici, and friend both of Piero de' Medici and Lorenzo. To explain Marsilio's influence it is necessary to recede a little into history. In 1439 Cosimo de' Medici succeeded in transferring the scene of the Great Council of the Church to Florence. At this conference representatives of the Western Church, centred in Rome, met those of the Eastern Church, centred in Constantinople, which was still Christian, for the purpose of discussing various matters, not the least of which was the protection of the Eastern Church against the Infidel. Not only was Constantinople continually threatened by the Turks, and in need of arms as well as sympathy, but the two branches of the Church were at enmity over a number of points. It was as much to heal these differences as to seek temporal aid that the Emperor John Palaeologus, the Patriarch of Constantinople, and a vast concourse of nobles, priests, and Greek scholars, arrived in Italy, and, after sojourning at Venice and Ferrara, moved on to Florence at the invitation of Cosimo. The Emperor resided in the Peruzzi palace, now no more, near S. Croce; the Patriarch of Constantinople lodged (and as it chanced, died, for he was very old) at the Ferrantini palace, now the Casa Vernaccia, in the Borgo Pinti; while Pope Eugenius was at the convent attached to S. Maria Novella. The meetings of the Council were held where we now stand–in the cathedral, whose dome had just been placed upon it all ready for them.

The Council failed in its purpose, and, as we know, Constantinople was lost some years later, and the great empire of which John Palaeologus was the last ruler ceased to be. That, however, at the moment is beside the mark. The interesting thing to us is that among the scholars who came from Constantinople, bringing with them numbers of manuscripts and systems of thought wholly new to the Florentines, was one Georgius Gemisthos, a Greek philosopher of much personal charm and comeliness, who talked a bland and beautiful Platonism that was extremely alluring not only to his youthful listeners but also to Cosimo himself. Gemisthos was, however, a Greek, and Cosimo was too busy a man in a city of enemies, or at any rate of the envious, to be able to do much more than extend his patronage to the old man and despatch emissaries to the East for more and more manuscripts; but discerning the allurements of the new gospel, Cosimo directed a Florentine enthusiast who knew Greek to spread the serene creed among his friends, who were all ripe for it, and this enthusiast was none other than a youthful scholar by name Marsilio Ficino, connected with S. Lorenzo, Cosimo's family church, and the son of Cosimo's own physician. To the young and ardent Marsilio, Plato became a god and Gemisthos not less than divine for bringing the tidings. He kept a lamp always burning before Plato's bust, and later founded the Platonic Academy, at which Plato's works were discussed, orations delivered, and new dialogues exchanged, between such keen minds as Marsilio, Pulci, Landini, Giovanni Cavalcanti, Leon Battista Alberti, the architect and scholar, Pico dell a Mirandola, the precocious disputant and aristocratic mystic, Poliziano, the tutor of Lorenzo's sons, and Lorenzo the Magnificent himself. It was thus from the Greek invasion of Florence that proceeded the stream of culture which is known as Humanism, and which, no doubt, in time, was so largely concerned in bringing about that indifference to spiritual things which, leading to general laxity and indulgence, filled Savonarola with despair.

I am not concerned to enter deeply into the subject of the Renaissance. But this must be said–that the new painting and sculpture, particularly the painting of Masaccio and the sculpture of Donatello, had shown the world that the human being could be made the measure of the Divine. The Madonna and Christ had been related to life. The new learning, by leading these keen Tuscan intellects, so eager for reasonableness, to the Greek philosophers who were so wise and so calm without any of the consolations of Christianity, naturally set them wondering if there were not a religion of Humanity that was perhaps a finer thing than the religion that required all the machinery and intrigue of Rome. And when, as the knowledge of Greek spread and the minute examination of documents ensued, it was found that Rome had not disdained forgery to gain her ends, a blow was struck against the Church from which it never recovered;–and how much of this was due to this Florentine Marsilio, sitting at the feet of the Greek Gemisthos, who came to Florence at the invitation of Cosimo de' Medici!

The cathedral glass, as I say, is mostly overladen with grime; but the circular windows in the dome seem to be magnificent in design. They are attributed to Ghiberti and Donatello, and are lovely in colour. The greens in particular are very striking. But the jewel of these circular windows of Florence is that by Ghiberti on the west wall of S. Croce.

And here I leave the Duomo, with the counsel to visitors to Florence to make a point of entering it every day–not, as so many Florentines do, in order to make a short cut from the Via Calzaioli to the Via de' Servi, and vice versâ, but to gather its spirit. It is different every hour in the day, and every hour the light enters it with new beauty.

CHAPTER III

The Duomo III: A Ceremony and a Museum

The Scoppio del Carro–The Pazzi beneficent–Holy Saturday's programme–April 6th, 1912–The flying palle–The nervous pyrotechnist–The influence of noon–A little sister of the Duomo–Donatello's cantoria–Luca della Robbia's cantoria.

In the last chapter we saw the Pazzi family as very black sheep, although there are plenty of students of Florentine history who hold that any attempt to rid Florence of the Medici was laudable. In this chapter we see them in a kindlier situation as benefactors to the city. For it happened that when Pazzo de' Pazzi, a founder of the house, was in the Holy Land during the First Crusade, it was his proud lot to set the Christian banner on the walls of Jerusalem, and, as a reward, Godfrey of Boulogne gave him some flints from the Holy Sepulchre. These he brought to Florence, and they are now preserved at SS. Apostoli, the little church in the Piazza del Limbo, off the Borgo SS. Apostoli, and every year the flints are used to kindle the fire needed for the right preservation of Easter Day. Gradually the ceremony enlarged until it became a spectacle indeed, which the Pazzi family for centuries controlled. After the Pazzi conspiracy they lost it and the Signoria took it over; but, on being pardoned, the Pazzi again resumed.

The Carro is a car containing explosives, and the Scoppio is its explosion. This car, after being drawn in procession through the streets by white oxen, is ignited by the sacred fire borne to it by a mechanical dove liberated at the high altar of the Duomo, and with its explosion Easter begins. There is still a Pazzi fund towards the expenses, but a few years ago the city became responsible for the whole proceedings, and the ceremony as it is now given, under civic management, known as the Scoppio del Cairo, is that which I saw on Holy Saturday last and am about to describe.

First, however, let me state what had happened before the proceedings opened in the Piazza del Duomo. At six o'clock mass began at SS. Apostoli, lasting for more than two hours. At its close the celebrant was handed a plate on which were the sacred flints, and these he struck with a steel in view of the congregation, thus igniting a taper. The candle, in an ancient copper porta fuoco surmounted by a dove, was then lighted, and the procession of priests started off for the cathedral with their precious flame, escorted by a civic guard and various standard bearers. Their route was the Piazza del Limbo, along the Borgo SS. Apostoli to the Via Por S. Maria and through the Vacchereccia to the Piazza della Signoria, the Via Condotta, the Via del Proconsolo, to the Duomo, through whose central doors they passed, depositing the sacred burden at the high altar. I should add that anyone on the route in charge of a street shrine had the right to stop the procession in order to take a light from it; while at SS. Apostoli women congregated with tapers and lanterns in the hope of getting these kindled from the sacred flame, in order to wash their babies or cook their food in water heated with the fire.

Meanwhile at seven o'clock the four oxen, which are kept in the Cascine all the year round and do no other work, had been harnessed to the car and had drawn it to the Piazza del Duomo, which was reached about nine. The oxen were then tethered by the Pisano doors of the Baptistery until needed again.

After some haggling on the night before, I had secured a seat on a balcony facing Ghiberti's first Baptistery doors, for eleven lire, and to this place I went at half-past ten. The piazza was then filling up, and at a quarter to eleven the trams running between the Cathedral and the Baptistery were stopped. In this space was the car. The present one, which dates from 1622, is more like a catafalque, and unless one sees it in motion, with the massive white oxen pulling it, one cannot believe in it as a vehicle at all. It is some thirty feet high, all black, with trumpery coloured-paper festoons (concealing fireworks) upon it: trumpery as only the Roman Catholic Church can contrive. It stood in front of the Duomo some four yards from the Baptistery gates in a line with the Duomo's central doors and the high altar. The doors were open, seats being placed on each side of the aisle the whole distance, and people making a solid avenue. Down this avenue were to come the clergy, and above it was to be stretched the line on which the dove was to travel from the altar, with the Pazzi fire, to ignite the car.

The space in front of the cathedral was cleared at about eleven, and cocked hats and red-striped trousers then became the most noticeable feature. The crowd was jolly and perhaps a little cynical; picture-postcard hawkers made most of the noise, and for some reason or other a forlorn peasant took this opportunity to offer for sale two equally forlorn hedgehogs. Each moment the concourse increased, for it is a fateful day and every one wants to know the issue: because, you see, if the dove runs true, lights the car, and returns, as a good dove should, to the altar ark, there will be a prosperous vintage and the pyrotechnist who controls the sacred bird's movements will receive his wages. But if the dove runs defectively and there is any hitch, every one is dismayed, for the harvest will be bad and the pyrotechnist will receive nothing. Once he was imprisoned when things went astray–and quite right too–but the Florentines have grown more lenient.

At about a quarter past eleven a procession of clergy emerged from the Duomo and crossed the space to the Baptistery. First, boys and youths in surplices. Then some scarlet hoods, waddling. Then purple hoods, and other colours, a little paunchier, waddling more, and lastly the archbishop, very sumptuous. All having disappeared into the Baptistery, through Ghiberti's second gates, which I never saw opened before, the dove's wire was stretched and fastened, a matter needing much care; and the crowds began to surge. The cocked hats and officers had the space all to themselves, with the car, the firemen, the pyrotechnist and the few privileged and very self-conscious civilians who were allowed inside.

A curious incident, which many years ago might have been magnified into a portent, occurred while the ecclesiastics were in the Artistry. Some one either bought and liberated several air balloons, or the string holding them was surreptitiously cut; but however it happened, the balls escaped and suddenly the crowd sent up a triumphant yell. At first I could see no reason for it, the Baptistery intervening, but then the balls swam into our ken and steadily floated over the cathedral out of sight amid tremendous satisfaction. And the portent? Well, as they moved against the blue sky they formed themselves into precisely the pattern of the palle on the Medici escutcheon. That is all. But think what that would have meant in the fifteenth century; the nods and frowns it would have occasioned; the dispersal of the Medici, the loss of power, and all the rest of it, that it would have presaged!

At about twenty to twelve the ecclesiastics returned and were swallowed up by the Duomo, and then excitement began to be acute. The pyrotechnist was not free from it; he fussed about nervously; he tested everything again and again; he crawled under the car and out of it; he talked to officials; he inspected and re-inspected. Photographers began to adjust their distances; the detached men in bowlers looked at their watches; the cocked hats drew nearer to the Duomo door. And then we heard a tearing noise. All eyes were turned to the great door, and out rushed the dove emitting a wake of sparks, entered the car and was out again on its homeward journey before one realized what had happened. And then the explosions began, and the bells–silent since Thursday–broke out. How many explosions there were I do not know; but they seemed to go on for ten minutes.

This is a great moment not only for the spectator but for all Florence, for in myriad rooms mothers have been waiting, with their babies on their knees, for the first clang of the belfries, because if a child's eyes are washed then it is unlikely ever to have weak sight, while if a baby takes its first steps to this accompaniment its legs will not be bowed.

At the last explosion the pyrotechnist, now a calm man once more and a proud one, approached the car, the firemen poured water on smouldering parts, and the work of clearing up began. Then came the patient oxen, their horns and hooves gilt, and great masses of flowers on their heads, and red cloths with the lily of Florence on it over their backs–much to be regretted since they obliterated their beautiful white skins–and slowly the car lumbered off, and, the cocked hats relenting, the crowd poured after it and the Scoppio del Carro was over.

The Duomo has a little sister in the shape of the Museo di Santa Maria del Fiore, or the Museo dell' Opera del Duomo, situated in the Piazza opposite the apse; and we should go there now. This museum, which is at once the smallest and, with the exception of the Natural History Museum, the cheapest of the Florentine museums, for it costs but half a lira, is notable for containing the two cantorie, or singing galleries, made for the cathedral, one by Donatello and one by Luca della Robbia. A cantoria by Donatello we shall soon see in its place in S. Lorenzo; but that, beautiful as it is, cannot compare with this one, with its procession of merry, dancing children, its massiveness and grace, its joyous ebullitions of gold mosaic and blue enamel. Both the cantorie–Donatello's, begun in 1433 and finished in 1439, and Luca's, begun in 1431 and finished in 1438–fulfilled their melodious functions in the Duomo until 1688, when they were ruthlessly cleared away to make room for large wooden balconies to be used in connexion with the nuptials of Ferdinand de' Medici and the Princess Violante of Bavaria. In the year 1688 taste was at a low ebb, and no one thought the deposed cantorie even worth preservation, so that they were broken up and occasionally levied upon for cornices and so forth. The fragments were collected and taken to the Bargello in the middle of the last century, and in 1883 Signer del Moro, the then architect of the Duomo (whose bust is in the courtyard of this museum), reconstructed them to the best of his ability in their present situation. It has to be remembered not only that, with the exception of the figures, the galleries are not as their artists made them, lacking many beautiful accessories, but that, as Vasari tells us, Donatello deliberately designed his for a dim light. None the less, they remain two of the most delightful works of the Renaissance and two of the rarest treasures of Florence.

The dancing boys behind the small pillars with their gold chequering, the brackets, and the urn of the cornice over the second pair of pillars from the right, are all that remain of Donatello's own handiwork. All else is new and conjectural. It is supposed that bronze heads of lions filled the two circular spaces between the brackets in the middle. But although the loss of the work as a whole is to be regretted, the dancing boys remain, to be for ever an inspiration and a pleasure. The Luca della Robbia cantoria opposite is not quite so triumphant a masterpiece, but from the point of view of suitability it is perhaps better. We can believe that Luca's children hymn the glory of the Lord, as indeed the inscription makes them, whereas Donatello's romp with a gladness that might easily be purely pagan. Luca's design is more formal, more conventional; Donatello's is rich and free and fluid with personality. The two end panels of Luca's are supplied in the cantoria by casts; the originals are on the wall below and may be carefully studied. The animation and fervour of these choristers are unforgettable.

It is well, while enjoying Donatello's work, to remember that Prato is only half an hour from Florence, and that there may be seen the open-air pulpit, built on the corner of the cathedral, which Donatello, with Michelozzo, his friend and colleague, made at the same time that the cantoria was in progress, and which in its relief of happy children is very similar, although not, I think, quite so remarkable. It lacks also the peculiarly naturalistic effect gained in the cantoria by setting the dancing boys behind the pillars, which undoubtedly, as comparison with the Luca shows, assists realism. The row of pillars attracts the eye first and the boys are thus thrown into a background which almost moves.

Although the cantorie dominate the museum they must not be allowed to overshadow all else. A marble relief of the Madonna and Children by Agostino di Duccio (1418-1481) must be sought for: it is No. 77 and the children are the merriest in Florence. Another memorable Madonna and Child is No. 94, by Pagno di Lapo Portigiani (1406-1470), who has interest for us in this place as being one of Donatello's assistants, very possibly on this very cantoria, and almost certainly on the Prato pulpit. Everything here, it must be remembered, has some association with the Duomo and was brought here for careful preservation and that whoever has fifty centimes might take pleasure in seeing it; but the great silver altar is from the Baptistery, and being made for that temple is naturally dedicated to the life of John the Baptist. Although much of it was the work of not the greatest modellers in the second half of the fourteenth century, three masters at least contributed later: Michelozzo adding the statue of the Baptist, Pollaiuolo the side relief depicting his birth, and Verrocchio that of his death, which is considered one of the most remarkable works of this sculptor, whom we are to find so richly represented at the Bargello. Before leaving this room, look for 100^3, an unknown terra-cotta of the Birth of Eve, which is both masterly and amusing, and 110^4, a very lovely intaglio in wood. I might add that among the few paintings, all very early, is a S. Sebastian in whose sacred body I counted no fewer than thirty arrows; which within my knowledge of pictures of this saint–not inconsiderable–is the highest number.

The next room is given to models and architectural plans and drawings connected with the cathedral, the most interesting thing being Brunelleschi's own model for the lantern. On the stairs are a series of fine bas-reliefs by Bandinelli and Giovanni dell' Opera from the old choir screen of the Duomo, and downstairs, among many other pieces of sculpture, is a bust of Brunelleschi from a death-mask and several beautiful della Robbia designs for lunettes over doors.

CHAPTER IV

THE Campanile and the Baptistery

A short way with Veronese critics–Giotto's missing spire–Donatello's holy men–Giotto as encyclopaedist–The seven and twenty reliefs–Ruskin in American–At the top of the tower–A sea of red roofs–The restful Baptistery–Historic stones–An ex-Pope's tomb–Andrea Pisano's doors–Ghiberti's first doors–Ghiberti's second doors–Michelangelo's praise–A gentleman artist.

It was in 1332, as I have said, that Giotto was made capo-maestro, and on July 18th, 1334, the first stone of his campanile was laid, the understanding being that the structure was to exceed "in magnificence, height, and excellence of workmanship" anything in the world. As some further indication of the glorious feeling of patriotism then animating the Florentines, it may be remarked that when a Veronese who happened to be in Florence ventured to suggest that the city was aiming rather too high, he was at once thrown into gaol, and, on being set free when his time was done, was shown the treasury as an object lesson. Of the wealth and purposefulness of Florence at that time, in spite of the disastrous bellicose period she had been passing through, Villani the historian, who wrote history as it was being made, gives an excellent account, which Macaulay summarizes in his vivid way. Thus:

"The revenue of the Republic amounted to three hundred thousand florins; a sum which, allowing for the depreciation of the precious metals, was at least equivalent to six hundred thousand pounds sterling; a larger sum than England and Ireland, two centuries ago, yielded to Elizabeth. The manufacture of wool alone employed two hundred factories and thirty thousand workmen. The cloth annually produced sold, at an average, for twelve hundred thousand florins; a sum fully equal in exchangeable value to two millions and a half of our money. Four hundred thousand florins were annually coined. Eighty banks conducted the commercial operations, not of Florence only but of all Europe. The transactions of these establishments were sometimes of a magnitude which may surprise even the contemporaries of the Barings and the Rothschilds. Two houses advanced to Edward III of England upwards of three hundred thousand marks, at a time when the mark contained more silver than fifty shillings of the present day, and when the value of silver was more than quadruple of what it now is. The city and its environs contained a hundred and seventy thousand children inhabitants. In the various schools about ten thousand children were taught to read; twelve hundred studied arithmetic; six hundred received a learned education."

Giotto died in 1386, and after his death, as I have said, Andrea Pisano came in for a while; to be followed by Talenti, who is said to have made considerable alterations in Giotto's design and to be responsible for the happy idea of increasing the height of the windows with the height of the tower and thus adding to the illusion of springing lightness. The topmost ones, so bold in size and so lovely with their spiral columns, almost seem to lift it.

The campanile to-day is 276 feet in height, and Giotto proposed to add to that a spire of 105 feet. The Florentines completed the façade of the cathedral in 1887 and are now spending enormous sums on the Medici chapel at S. Lorenzo; why should they not one day carry out their greatest artist's intention?

The campanile as a structure had been finished in 1387, but not for many years did it receive its statues, of which something must be said, although it is impossible to get more than a vague idea of them, so high are they. A captive balloon should be arranged for the use of visitors. Those by Donatello, on the Baptistery side, are the most remarkable. The first of these–that nearest to the cathedral and the most striking as seen from the distant earth–is called John the Baptist, always a favourite subject with this sculptor, who, since he more than any at that thoughtful time endeavoured to discover and disclose the secret of character, is curiously unfortunate in the accident that has fastened names to these figures. This John, for example, bears no relation to his other Baptists; nor does the next figure represent David, as is generally supposed, but owes that error to the circumstance that when the David that originally stood here was moved to the north side, the old plinth bearing his name was left behind. This famous figure is stated by Vasari to be a portrait of a Florentine merchant named Barduccio Cherichini, and for centuries it has been known as Il Zuccone (or pumpkin) from its baldness. Donatello, according to Vasari, had a particular liking for the work, so much that he used to swear by it; while, when engaged upon it, he is said to have so believed in its reality as to exclaim, "Speak, speak! or may a dysentery seize thee!" It is now generally considered to represent Job, and we cannot too much regret the impossibility of getting near enough to study it. Next is the Jeremiah, which, according to Vasari, was a portrait of another Florentine, but which, since he bears his name on a scroll, may none the less be taken to realize the sculptor's idea of Jeremiah. It is (according to the photographs) a fine piece of rugged vivacity, and the head is absolutely that of a real man. On the opposite side of the tower is the magnificent Abraham's sacrifice from the same strong hand, and by it Habakkuk, who is no less near life than the Jeremiah and Job, but a very different type. At both Or San Michele and the Bargello we are to find Donatello perhaps in a finer mood than here, and comfortably visible.

For most visitors to Florence and all disciples of Ruskin, the chief interest of the campanile ("The Shepherd's Tower" as he calls it) is the series of twenty-seven reliefs illustrating the history of the world and the progress of mankind, which are to be seen round the base, the design, it is supposed, of Giotto, executed by Andrea Pisano and Luca della Robbia. To Andrea are given all those on the west (7), south (7), east (5), and the two eastern ones on the north; to Luca the remaining five on the north. Ruskin's fascinating analysis of these reliefs should most certainly be read (without a total forgetfulness of the shepherd's other activities as a painter, architect, humorist, and friend of princes and poets), but equally certainly not in the American pirated edition which the Florentine booksellers are so ready (to their shame) to sell you. Only Ruskin in his best mood of fury could begin to do justice to the misspellings and mispunctuations of this terrible production.

Ruskin, I may say, believes several of the carvings to be from Giotto's own chisel as well as design, but other and more modern authorities disagree, although opinion now inclines to the belief that the designs for Pisano's Baptistery doors are also his. Such thoroughness and ingenuity were all in Giotto's way, and they certainly suggest his active mind. The campanile series begins at the west side with the creation of man. Among the most attractive are, I think, those devoted to agriculture, with the spirited oxen, to astronomy, to architecture, to weaving, and to pottery. Giotto was even so thorough as to give one relief to the conquest of the air; and he makes Noah most satisfactorily drunk. Note also the Florentine fleur-de-lis round the base of the tower. Every fleur-de-lis in Florence is beautiful–even those on advertisements and fire-plugs–but few are more beautiful than these.

I climbed the campanile one fine morning–417 steps from the ground–and was well repaid; but I think it is wiser to ascend the tower of the Palazzo Vecchio, because one is higher there and, since the bulk of the dome, which intrudes from the campanile, is avoided, one has a better all-round view. Florence seen from this eminence is very red–so uniformly so that many towers rise against it almost indistinguishably, particularly the Bargello's and the Badia's. One sees at once how few straight streets there are–the Ricasoli standing out among them as the exception; and one realizes how the city has developed outside, with its boulevards where the walls once were, leaving the gates isolated, and its cincture of factories. The occasional glimpses of cloisters and verdure among the red are very pleasant. One of the objects cut off by the cathedral dome is the English cemetery, but the modern Jewish temple stands out as noticeably almost as any of the ancient buildings. The Pitti looks like nothing but a barracks and the Porta Ferdinando has prominence which it gets from no other point. The roof of the Mercato Centrale is the ugliest thing in the view. While I was there the midday gun from the Boboli fortress was fired, instantly having its punctual double effect of sending all the pigeons up in a grey cloud of simulated alarm and starting every bell in the city.

Those wishing to make either the campanile or Duomo ascents must remember to do it early. The closing hour for the day being twelve, no one is allowed to start up after about a quarter past eleven: a very foolish arrangement, since Florence and the surrounding Apennines under a slanting sun are more beautiful than in the morning glare, and the ascent would be less fatiguing. As it was, on descending, after being so long at the top, I was severely reprimanded by the custodian, who had previously marked me down as a barbarian for refusing his offer of field-glasses. But the Palazzo Vecchio tower is open till five.

The Baptistery is the beautiful octagonal building opposite the cathedral, and once the cathedral itself. It dates from the seventh or eighth century, but as we see it now is a product chiefly of the thirteenth. The bronze doors opposite the Via Calzaioli are open every day, a circumstance which visitors, baffled by the two sets of Ghiberti doors always so firmly closed, are apt to overlook. All children born in Florence are still baptized here, and I watched one afternoon an old priest at the task, a tiny Florentine being brought in to receive the name of Tosca, which she did with less distaste than most, considering how thorough was his sprinkling. The Baptistery is rich in colour both without and within. The floor alone is a marvel of intricate inlaying, including the signs of the zodiac and a gnomic sentence which reads the same backwards and forwards–"En gire torte sol ciclos et roterigne". On this very pavement Dante, who called the church his "beautiful San Giovanni," has walked. Over the altar is a gigantic and primitive Christ in mosaic, more splendid than spiritual. The mosaics in the recesses of the clerestory–grey and white–are the most soft and lovely of all. I believe the Baptistery is the most restful place in Florence; and this is rather odd considering that it is all marble and mosaic patterns. But its shape is very soothing, and age has given it a quality of its own, and there is just that touch of barbarism about it such as one gets in Byzantine buildings to lend it a peculiar character here.

The most notable sculpture in the Baptistery is the tomb of the ex-Pope John XXIII, whose licentiousness was such that there was nothing for it but to depose and imprison him. He had, however, much money, and on his liberation he settled in Florence, presented a true finger of John the Baptist to the Baptistery, and arranged in return for his bones to repose in that sanctuary. One of his executors was that Niccolò da Uzzano, the head of the noble faction in the city, whose coloured bust by Donatello is in the Bargello. The tomb is exceedingly fine, the work of Donatello and his partner Michelozzo, who were engaged to make it by Giovanni de' Medici, the ex-pontiff's friend, and the father of the great Cosimo. The design is all Donatello's, and his the recumbent cleric, lying very naturally, hardly as if dead at all, a little on one side, so that his face is seen nearly full, the three figures beneath are Michelozzo's; but Donatello probably carved the seated angels who display the scroll which bears the dead Pope's name. The Madonna and Child above are by Donatello's assistant, Pagno di Lapo Portigiani, a pretty relief by whom we saw in the Museum of the Cathedral. Being in red stone, and very dusty, like Ghiberti's doors (which want the hose regularly), the lines of the tomb are much impaired. Donatello is also represented here by a Mary Magdalene in wood, on an altar at the left of the entrance door, very powerful and poignant.

In the ordinary way, when visitors to Florence speak of the Baptistery doors they mean those opposite the Duomo, and when they go to the Bargello and look at the designs made by Ghiberti and Brunelleschi in competition, they think that the competition was for those. But that is wrong. Ghiberti won his spurs with the doors on the north side, at which comparatively few persons look. The famous doors opposite the Duomo were commissioned many years later, when his genius was acknowledged and when he had become so accomplished as to do what he liked with his medium. Before, however, coming to Ghiberti, we ought to look at the work of an early predecessor but for whom there might have been no Ghiberti at all; for while Ghiberti was at work with his assistants on these north doors, between 1403 and 1424, the place which they occupy was filled by those executed seventy years earlier by Andrea Pisano (1270-1348), possibly from Giotto's designs, which are now at the south entrance, opposite the charming little loggia at the corner of the Via Calzaioli, called the Bigallo. These represent twenty scenes in the life of S. John the Baptist, and below them are eight figures of cardinal and Christian virtues, and they employed their sculptor from 1330 to 1336. They have three claims to notice: as being admirably simple and vigorous in themselves; as having influenced all later workers in this medium, and particularly Ghiberti and Donatello; and as being the bronze work of the sculptor of certain of the stone scenes round the base of Giotto's campanile. The panel in which the Baptist is seen up to his waist in the water is surely the very last word in audacity in bronze. Ghiberti was charged with making bronze do things that it was ill fitted for; but I do not know that even he moulded water–and transparent water–from it.

The year 1399 is one of the most notable in the history of modern art, since it was then that the competition for the Baptistery gates was made public, this announcement being the spring from which many rivers flowed. In that year Lorenzo Ghiberti, a young goldsmith assisting his father, was twenty-one, and Filippo Brunelleschi, another goldsmith, was twenty-two, while Giotto had been dead sixty-three years and the impulse he had given to painting had almost worked itself out. The new doors were to be of the same shape and size as those by Andrea Pisano, which were already getting on for seventy years old, and candidates were invited to make a specimen relief to scale, representing the interrupted sacrifice of Isaac, although the subject-matter of the doors was to be the Life of S. John the Baptist. Among the judges was that Florentine banker whose name was beginning to be known in the city as a synonym for philanthropy, enlightenment, and sagacity, Giovanni de' Medici. In 1401 the specimens were ready, and after much deliberation as to which was the better, Ghiberti's or Brunelleschi's–assisted, some say, by Brunelleschi's own advice in favour of his rival–the award was given to Ghiberti, and he was instructed to proceed with his task; while Brunelleschi, as we have seen, being a man of determined ambition, left for Rome to study architecture, having made up his mind to be second to no one in whichever of the arts and crafts he decided to pursue. Here then was the first result of the competition–that it turned Brunelleschi to architecture.

Ghiberti began seriously in 1408 and continued till 1424, when the doors were finished; but, in order to carry out the work, he required assistance in casting and so forth, and for that purpose engaged among others a sculptor named Donatello (born in 1386), a younger sculptor named Luca della Robbia (born in 1400), and a gigantic young painter called Masaccio (born in 1401), each of whom was destined, taking fire no doubt from Ghiberti and his fine free way, to be a powerful innovator–Donatello (apart from other and rarer achievements) being the first sculptor since antiquity to place a statue on a pedestal around which observers could walk; Masaccio being the first painter to make pictures in the modern use of the term, with men and women of flesh and blood in them, as distinguished from decorative saints, and to be by example the instructor of all the greatest masters, from his pupil Lippo Lippi to Leonardo and Michelangelo; and Luca della Robbia being the inspired discoverer of an inexpensive means of glazing terra-cotta so that his beautiful and radiant Madonnas could be brought within the purchasing means of the poorest congregation in Italy. These alone are remarkable enough results, but when we recollect also that Brunelleschi's defeat led to the building of the cathedral dome, the significance of the event becomes the more extraordinary.

The doors, as I say, were finished in 1424, after twenty-one years' labour, and the Signoria left the Palazzo Vecchio in procession to see their installation. In the number and shape of the panels Pisano set the standard, but Ghiberti's work resembled that of his predecessor very little in other ways, for he had a mind of domestic sweetness without austerity and he was interested in making everything as easy and fluid and beautiful as might be. His thoroughness recalls Giotto in certain of his frescoes. The impression left by Pisano's doors is akin to that left by reading the New Testament; but Ghiberti makes everything happier than that. Two scenes–both on the level of the eye–I particularly like: the "Annunciation," with its little, lithe, reluctant Virgin, and the "Adoration". The border of the Pisano doors is, I think, finer than that of Ghiberti's; but it is a later work.

Looking at them even now, with eyes that remember so much of the best art that followed them and took inspiration from them, we can understand the better how delighted Florence must have been with this new picture gallery and how the doors were besieged by sightseers. But greater still was to come. Ghiberti at once received the commission to make two more doors on his own scale for the south side of the Baptistery, and in 1425 he had begun on them. These were not finished until 1452, so that Ghiberti, then a man of seventy-four, had given practically his whole life to the making of four bronze doors. It is true that he did a few other things besides, such as the casket of S. Zenobius in the Duomo, and the Baptist and S. Matthew for Or San Michele; but he may be said justly to live by his doors, and particularly by the second pair, although it was the first pair that had the greater effect on his contemporaries and followers.

Among his assistants on these were Antonio Pollaiuolo (born in 1429), who designed the quail in the left border, and Paolo Uccello (born in 1397), both destined to be men of influence. The bald head on the right door is a portrait of Ghiberti; that of the old man on the left is his father, who helped him to polish the original competition plaque. Although commissioned for the south side they were placed where they now are, on the east, as being most worthy of the position of honour, and Pisano's doors, which used to be here, were moved to the south, where they now are.

On Ghiberti's workshop opposite S. Maria Nuova, in the Via Bufalini, the memorial tablet mentions Michelangelo's praise–that these doors were beautiful enough to be the Gates of Paradise. After that what is an ordinary person to say? That they are lovely is a commonplace. But they are more. They are so sensitive; bronze, the medium which Horace has called, by implication, the most durable of all, has become in Ghiberti's hands almost as soft as wax and tender as flesh. It does all he asks; it almost moves; every trace of sternness has vanished from it. Nothing in plastic art that we have ever seen or shall see is more easy and ingratiating than these almost living pictures.

Before them there is steadily a little knot of admirers, and on Sundays you may always see country people explaining the panels to each other. Every one has his favourite among these fascinating Biblical scenes, and mine are Cain and Abel, with the ploughing, and Abraham and Isaac, with its row of fir trees. It has been explained by the purists that the sculptor stretched the bounds of plastic art too far and made bronze paint pictures; but most persons will agree to ignore that. Of the charm of Ghiberti's mind the border gives further evidence, with its fruits and foliage, birds and woodland creatures, so true to life, and here fixed for all time, so naturally, that if these animals should ever (as is not unlikely in Italy where every one has a gun and shoots at his pleasure) become extinct, they could be created again from these designs.

Ghiberti, who enjoyed great honour in his life and a considerable salary as joint architect of the dome with Brunelleschi, died three years after the completion of the second doors and was buried in S. Croce. His place in Florentine art is unique and glorious.

The broken porphyry pillars by these second doors were a gift from Pisa to Florence in recognition of Florence's watchfulness over Pisa while the Pisans were away subduing the Balearic islanders.

The bronze group over Ghiberti's first doors, representing John the Baptist preaching between a Pharisee and a Levite, are the work (either alone or assisted by his master Leonardo da Vinci) of an interesting Florentine sculptor, Giovanni Francesco Rustici (1474-1554), who was remarkable among the artists of his time in being what we should call an amateur, having a competence of his own and the manners of a patron. Placing himself under Verrocchio, he became closely attached to Leonardo, a fellow-pupil, and made him his model rather than the older man. He took his art lightly, and lived, in Vasari's phrase, "free from care," having such beguilements as a tame menagerie (Leonardo, it will be remembered, loved animals too and had a habit of buying small caged birds in order to set them free), and two or three dining clubs, the members of which vied with each other in devising curious and exotic dishes. Andrea del Sarto, for example, once brought as his contribution to the feast a model of this very church we are studying, the Baptistery, of which the floor was constructed of jelly, the pillars of sausages, and the choir desk of cold veal, while the choristers were roast thrushes. Rustici further paved the way to a life free from care by appointing a steward of his estate whose duty it was to see that his money-box, to which he went whenever he wanted anything, always had money in it. This box he never locked, having learned that he need fear no robbery by once leaving his cloak for two days under a bush and then finding it again. "This world," he exclaimed, "is too good: it will not last." Among his pets were a porcupine trained to prick the legs of his guests under the table "so that they drew them in quickly"; a raven that spoke like a human being; an eagle, and many snakes. He also studied necromancy, the better to frighten his apprentices. He left Florence in 1528, after the Medici expulsion, and, like Leonardo, took service with Francis the First. He died at the age of eighty.

I had an hour and more exactly opposite the Rustici group, on the same level, while waiting for the Scoppio del Carro, and I find it easy to believe that Leonardo himself had a hand in the work. The figure of the Baptist is superb, the attitude of his listeners masterly.

CHAPTER V

THE Riccardi Palace and the Medici

An evasion of history–"Il Caparra"–The Gozzoli frescoes–Giovanni de' Medici (di Bicci)–Cosimo de' Medici–The first banishment–Piero de' Medici–Lorenzo de' Medici–Piero di Lorenzo de' Medici–The second banishment–Giuliano di Lorenzo de' Medici–Leo X–Lorenzo di Piero di Lorenzo de' Medici–Clement VII–Third banishment of the Medici–The siege of Florence–Alessandro de' Medici–Ippolito de' Medici–Lorenzino de' Medici–Giovanni delle Bande Nere–Cosimo I–The Grand Dukes.

The natural step from the Baptistery would be to the Uffizi. But for us not yet; because in order to understand Florence, and particularly the Florence that existed between the extreme dates that I have chosen as containing the fascinating period–namely 1296, when the Duomo was begun, and 1564, when Michelangelo died–one must understand who and what the Medici were.

While I have been enjoying the pleasant task of writing this book–which has been more agreeable than any literary work I have ever done–I have continually been conscious of a plaintive voice at my shoulder, proceeding from one of the vigilant and embarrassing imps who sit there and do duty as conscience, inquiring if the time is not about ripe for introducing that historical sketch of Florence without which no account such as this can be rightly understood. And ever I have replied with words of a soothing and procrastinating nature. But now that we are face to face with the Medici family, in their very house, I am conscious that the occasion for that historical sketch is here indeed, and equally I am conscious of being quite incapable of supplying it. For the history of Florence between, say the birth of Giotto or Dante and the return of Cosimo de' Medici from exile, when the absolute Medici rule began, is so turbulent, crowded, and complex that it would require the whole of this volume to describe it. The changes in the government of the city would alone occupy a good third, so constant and complicated were they. I should have to explain the Guelphs and the Ghibellines, the Neri and the Bianchi, the Guilds and the Priors, the gonfalonieri and the podesta, the secondo popolo and the buonuomini.

Rather than do this imperfectly I have chosen to do it not at all; and the curious must resort to historians proper. But there is at the end of the volume a table of the chief dates in Florentine and European history in the period chosen, together with births and deaths of artists and poets and other important persons, so that a bird's-eye view of the progress of affairs can be quickly gained, while in this chapter I offer an outline of the great family of rulers of Florence who made the little city an aesthetic lawgiver to the world and with whom her later fame, good or ill, is indissolubly united. For the rest, is there not the library?

The Medici, once so powerful and stimulating, are still ever in the background of Florence as one wanders hither and thither. They are behind many of the best pictures and most of the best statues. Their escutcheon is everywhere. I ought, I believe, to have made them the subject of my first chapter. But since I did not, let us without further delay turn to the Via Cavour, which runs away to the north from the Baptistery, being a continuation of the Via de' Martelli, and pause at the massive and dignified palace at the first corner on the left. For that is the Medici's home; and afterwards we will step into S. Lorenzo and see the church which Brunelleschi and Donatello made beautiful and Michelangelo wonderful that the Medici might lie there.

Visitors go to the Riccardi palace rather to see Gozzoli's frescoes than anything else; and indeed apart from the noble solid Renaissance architecture of Michelozzo there is not much else to see. In the courtyard are certain fragments of antique sculpture arranged against the walls, and a sarcophagus is shown in which an early member of the family, Guccio de' Medici, who was gonfalonier in 1299, once reposed. There too are Donatello's eight medallions, but they are not very interesting, being only enlarged copies of old medals and cameos and not notable for his own characteristics.

Hence it is that, after Gozzoli, by far the most interesting part of this building is its associations. For here lived Cosimo de' Medici, whose building of the palace was interrupted by his banishment as a citizen of dangerous ambition; here lived Piero de' Medici, for whom Gozzoli worked; here was born and here lived Lorenzo the Magnificent. To this palace came the Pazzi conspirators to lure Giuliano to the Duomo and his doom. Here did Charles VIII–Savonarola's "Flagellum Dei"–lodge and loot, and it was here that Capponi frightened him with the threat of the Florentine bells; hither came in 1494 the fickle and terrible Florentine mob, always passionate in its pursuit of change and excitement, and now inflamed by the sermons of Savonarola, to destroy the priceless manuscripts and works of art; here was brought up for a year or so the little Catherine de' Medici, and next door was the house in which Alessandro de' Medici was murdered.

It was in the seventeenth century that the palace passed to the Riccardi family, who made many additions. A century later Florence acquired it, and to-day it is the seat of the Prefect of the city. Cosimo's original building was smaller; but much of it remains untouched. The exquisite cornice is Michelozzo's original, and the courtyard has merely lost its statues, among which are Donatello's Judith, now in the Loggia de' Lanzi, and his bronze David, now in the Bargello, while Verrocchio's David was probably on the stairs. The escutcheon on the corner of the house gives us the period of its erection. The seven plain balls proclaim it Cosimo's. Each of the Medici sported these palle, although each had also his private crest. Under Giovanni, Cosimo's father, the balls were eight in number; under Cosimo, seven; under Piero, seven, with the fleur-de-lis of France on the uppermost, given him by Louis XI; under Lorenzo, six; and as one walks about Florence one can approximately fix the date of a building by remembering these changes. How many times they occur on the façades of Florence and its vicinity, probably no one could say; but they are everywhere. The French wits, who were amused to derive Catherine de' Medici from a family of apothecaries, called them pills.

The beautiful lantern at the corner was added by Lorenzo and was the work of an odd ironsmith in Florence for whom he had a great liking–Niccolò Grosso. For Lorenzo had all that delight in character which belongs so often to the born patron and usually to the born connoisseur. This Grosso was a man of humorous independence and bluntness. He had the admirable custom of carrying out his commissions in the order in which they arrived, so that if he was at work upon a set of fire-irons for a poor client, not even Lorenzo himself (who as a matter of fact often tried) could induce him to turn to something more lucrative. The rich who cannot wait he forced to wait. Grosso also always insisted upon something in advance and payment on delivery, and pleasantly described his workshop as being the Sign of the Burning Books,–since if his books were burnt how could he enter a debt? This rule earned for him from Lorenzo the nickname of "Il Caparra" (earnest money). Another of Grosso's eccentricities was to refuse to work for Jews.

Within the palace, up stairs, is the little chapel which Gozzoli made so gay and fascinating that it is probably the very gem among the private chapels of the world. Here not only did the Medici perform their devotions–Lorenzo's corner seat is still shown, and anyone may sit in it–but their splendour and taste are reflected on the walls. Cosimo, as we shall see when we reach S. Marco, invited Fra Angelico to paint upon the walls of that convent sweet and simple frescoes to the glory of God. Piero employed Fra Angelico's pupil, Benozzo Gozzoli to decorate this chapel.

In the year 1439, as chapter II related, through the instrumentality of Cosimo a great episcopal Council was held at Florence, at which John Palaeologus, Emperor of the East, met Pope Eugenius IV. In that year Cosimo's son Piero was twenty-three, and Gozzoli nineteen, and probably upon both, but certainly on the young artist, such pomp and splendour and gorgeousness of costume as then were visible in Florence made a deep impression. When therefore Piero, after becoming head of the family, decided to decorate the chapel with a procession of Magi, it is not surprising that the painter should recall this historic occasion. We thus get the pageantry of the East with more than common realism, while the portraits, or at any rate representations, of the Patriarch of Constantinople (the first king) and the Emperor (the second king) are here, together with those of certain Medici, for the youthful third king is none other than Piero's eldest son Lorenzo. Among their followers are (the third on the left) Cosimo de' Medici, who is included as among the living, although, like the Patriarch of Constantinople, he was dead, and his brother Lorenzo (the middle one of the three), whose existence is forgotten so completely until the accession of Cosimo I, in 1537, brings his branch of the family into power; while on the right is Piero de' Medici himself. Piero's second son Giuliano is on the white horse, preceded by a negro carrying his bow. The head immediately above Giuliano I do not know, but that one a little to the left above it is Gozzoli's own. Among the throng are men of learning who either came to Florence from the East or Florentines who assimilated their philosophy–such as Georgius Gemisthos, Marsilio Ficino, and perhaps certain painters among them, all protégés of Cosimo and Piero, and all makers of the Renaissance.

The assemblage alone, apart altogether from any beauty and charm that the painting possesses, makes these frescoes valuable. But the painting is a delight. We have a pretty Gozzoli in our National Gallery–No. 283–but it gives no indication of the ripeness and richness and incident of this work; while the famous Biblical series in the Campo Santo of Pisa has so largely perished as to be scarcely evidence to his colour. The first impression made by the Medici frescoes is their sumptuousness. When Gozzoli painted–if the story be true–he had only candle light: the window over the altar is new. But think of candle light being all the illumination of these walls as the painter worked! A new door and window have also been cut in the wall opposite the altar close to the three daughters of Piero, by vandal hands; and "Bruta, bruta!" says the guardian, very rightly.

The landscape behind the procession is hardly less interesting than the procession itself; but it is when we come to the meadows of paradise, with the angels and roses, the cypresses and birds, in the two chancel scenes, that this side of Gozzoli's art is most fascinating. He has travelled a long way from his master Fra Angelico here: the heaven is of the visible rather than the invisible eye; sense is present as well as the rapturous spirit. The little Medici who endured the tedium of the services here are to be felicitated with upon such an adorable presentment of glory. With plenty of altar candles the sight of these gardens of the blest must have beguiled many a mass. Thinking here in England upon the Medici chapel, I find that the impression it has left upon me is chiefly cypresses–cypresses black and comely, disposed by a master hand, with a glint of gold among them.

The picture that was over the altar has gone. It was a Lippo Lippi and is now in Berlin.

The first of the Medici family to rise to the highest power was Giovanni d'Averardo de' Medici (known as Giovanni di Bicci), 1360-1429, who, a wealthy banker living in what is now the Piazza del Duomo, was well known for his philanthropy and interest in the welfare of the Florentines, but does not come much into public notice until 1401, when he was appointed one of the judges in the Baptistery door competition. He was a retiring, watchful man. Whether he was personally ambitious is not too evident, but he was opposed to tyranny and was the steady foe of the Albizzi faction, who at that time were endeavouring to obtain supreme power in Florentine affairs. In 1419

Giovanni increased his popularity by founding the Spedale degli Innocenti, and in 1421 he was elected gonfalonier, or, as we might now say, President of the Republic. In this capacity he made his position secure and reduced the nobles (chief of whom was Niccolò da Uzzano) to political weakness. Giovanni died in 1429, leaving one son, Cosimo, aged forty, a second, Lorenzo, aged thirtyfour, a fragrant memory and an immense fortune.

To Lorenzo, who remained a private citizen, we shall return in time; it is Cosimo (1389-1464) with whom we are now concerned. Cosimo de' Medici was a man of great mental and practical ability: he had been educated as well as possible; he had a passion both for art and letters; he inherited his father's financial ability and generosity, while he added to these gifts a certain genius for the management of men. One of the first things that Cosimo did after his father's death was to begin the palace where we now are, rejecting a plan by Brunelleschi as too splendid, and choosing instead one by Michelozzo, the partner of Donatello, two artists who remained his personal friends through life. Cosimo selected this site, in what was then the Via Larga but is now the Via Cavour, partly because his father had once lived there, and partly because it was close to S. Lorenzo, which his father, with six other families, had begun to rebuild, a work he intended himself to carry on.

The palace was begun in 1430 abd was still in progress in 1433 when the Albizzi, who had always viewed the rise of the Medici family with apprehension and misgiving, and were now strengthened by the death of Niccolò da Uzzano, who, though powerful, had been a very cautious and temperate adviser, succeeded in getting a majority in the Signoria and passing a sentence of banishment on the whole Medici tribe as being too rich and ambitious to be good citizens of a simple and frugal Republic. Cosimo therefore, after some days of imprisonment in the tower of the Palazzo Vecchio, during which he expected execution at any moment, left Florence for Venice, taking his architect with him. In 1434, however, the Florentines, realizing that under the Albizzi they were losing their independence, and what was to be a democracy was become an oligarchy, revolted, and Cosimo was recalled, and, like his father, was elected gonfalonier. With this recall began his long supremacy; for he returned like a king and like a king remained, quickly establishing himself as the leading man in the city, the power behind the Signoria. Not only did he never lose that position, but he made it so naturally his own that when he died he was able to transmit it to his son.

Cosimo de' Medici was, I think, the wisest and best ruler that Florence ever had and ranks high among the rulers that any state ever had. But he changed the Florentines from an independent people to a dependent one. In his capacity of Father of his Country he saw to it that his children lost their proud spirit. He had to be absolute; and this end he achieved in many ways, but chiefly by his wealth, which made it possible to break the rich rebel and to enslave the poor. His greatest asset–next his wealth–was his knowledge of the Florentine character. To know anything of this capricious, fickle, turbulent folk even after the event was in itself a task of such magnitude that almost no one else had compassed it; but Cosimo did more, he knew what they were likely to do. By this knowledge, together with his riches, his craft, his tact, his business ramifications as an international banker, his open-handedness and air of personal simplicity, Cosimo made himself a power. For Florence could he not do enough. By inviting the Pope and the Greek Emperor to meet there he gave it great political importance, and incidentally brought about the New Learning. He established the Platonic Academy and formed the first public library in the west. He rebuilt and endowed the monastery of S. Marco. He built and rebuilt other churches. He gave Donatello a free hand in sculpture and Fra Lippo Lippi and Fra Angelico in painting. He distributed altogether in charity and churches four hundred thousand of those golden coins which were invented by Florence and named florins after her–a sum equal to a million pounds of to-day. In every direction one comes upon traces of his generosity and thoroughness. After his death it was decided that as Pater Patriae, or Father of his Country, he should be for ever known.

Cosimo died in 1464, leaving an invalid son, Piero, aged forty-eight, known for his almost continuous gout as Il Gottoso. Giovanni and Cosimo had

had to work for their power; Piero stepped naturally into it, although almost immediately he had to deal with a plot–the first for thirty years–to ruin the Medici prestige, the leader of which was that Luca Pitti who began the Pitti palace in order to have a better house than the Medici. The plot failed, not a little owing to young Lorenzo de' Medici's address, and the remaining few years of Piero's life were tranquil. He was a quiet, kindly man with the traditional family love of the arts, and it was for him that Gozzoli worked. He died in 1469, leaving two sons, Lorenzo (1449-1492) and Giuliano (1453-1478).

Lorenzo had been brought up as the future leading citizen of Florence: he had every advantage of education and environment, and was rich in the aristocratic spirit which often blossoms most richly in the second or third generation of wealthy business families. Giovanni had been a banker before everything, Cosimo an administrator, Piero a faithful inheritor of his father's wishes; it was left for Lorenzo to be the first poet and natural prince of the Medici blood. Lorenzo continued to bank but mismanaged the work and lost heavily; while his poetical tendencies no doubt distracted his attention generally from affairs. Yet such was his sympathetic understanding and his native splendour and gift of leadership that he could not but be at the head of everything, the first to be consulted and ingratiated. Not only was he the first Medici poet but the first of the family to marry not for love but for policy, and that too was a sign of decadence.

Lorenzo came into power when only twenty, and at the age of forty-two he was dead, but in the interval, by his interest in every kind of intellectual and artistic activity, by his passion for the greatness and glory of Florence, he made for himself a name that must always connote liberality, splendour, and enlightenment. But it is beyond question that under Lorenzo the Florentines changed deeply and for the worse. The old thrift and simplicity gave way to extravagance and ostentation; the old faith gave way too, but that was not wholly the effect of Lorenzo's natural inclination towards Platonic philosophy, fostered by his tutor Marsilio Ficino and his friends Poliziano and

Pico della Mirandola, but was due in no small measure also to the hostility of Pope Sixtus, which culminated in the Pazzi Conspiracy of 1478 and the murder of Giuliano. Looking at the history of Florence from our present vantage-point we can see that although under Lorenzo the Magnificent she was the centre of the world's culture and distinction, there was behind this dazzling front no seriousness of purpose. She was in short enjoying the fruits of her labours as though the time of rest had come; and this when strenuousness was more than ever important. Lorenzo carried on every good work of his father and grandfather (he spent £65,000 a year in books alone) and was as jealous of Florentine interests; but he was also "The Magnificent," and in that lay the peril. Florence could do with wealth and power, but magnificence went to her head.

Lorenzo died in 1492, leaving three sons, of whom the eldest, Piero (1471-1503), succeeded him. Never was such a decadence. In a moment the Medici prestige, which had been steadily growing under Cosimo, Piero, and Lorenzo until it was world famous, crumbled to dust. Piero was a coarse-minded, pleasure-loving youth–"The Headstrong" his father had called him–whose one idea of power was to be sensual and tyrannical; and the enemies of Florence and of Italy took advantage of this fact. Savonarola's sermons had paved the way from within too. In 1494 Charles VIII of France marched into Italy; Piero pulled himself together and visited the king to make terms for Florence, but made such terms that on returning to the city he found an order of banishment and obeyed it. On November 9th, 1494, he and his family were expelled, and the mob, forgetting so quickly all that they owed to the Medici who had gone before, rushed to this beautiful palace and looted it. The losses that art and learning sustained in a few hours can never be estimated. A certain number of treasures were subsequently collected again, such as Donatello's David and Verrocchio's David, while Donatello's Judith was removed to the Palazzo Vecchio, where an inscription was placed upon it saying that her short way with Holofernes was a warning to all traitors; but priceless pictures, sculpture, and MSS. were ruthlessly demolished.

In the chapter on S. Marco we shall read of what experiments in government the Florentines substituted for that of the Medici, Savonarola for a while being at the head of the government, although only for a brief period which ended amid an orgy of lawlessness; and then, after a restless period of eighteen years, in which Florence had every claw cut and was weakened also by dissension, the Medici returned–the change being the work of Lorenzo's second son, Giovanni de' Medici, who on the eve of becoming Pope Leo X procured their reinstatement, thus justifying the wisdom of his father in placing him in the Church. Piero having been drowned long since, his admirable but ill-starred brother Giuliano, Duke of Nemours, now thirty-three, assumed the control, always under Leo X; while their cousin, Giulio, also a Churchman, and the natural son of the murdered Giuliano, was busy, behind the scenes, with the family fortunes.

Giuliano lived only till 1516 and was succeeded by his nephew Lorenzo, Duke of Urbino, a son of Peiro, a young man of no more political use than his father, and one who quickly became almost equally unpopular. Things indeed were going so badly that Leo X sent Giulio de' Medici (now a cardinal) from Rome to straighten them out, and by some sensible repeals he succeeded in allaying a little of the bitterness in the city. Lorenzo had one daughter, born in this palace, who was destined to make history–Catherine de' Medici–and no son. When therefore he died in 1519, at the age of twenty-seven, after a life of vicious selfishness (which, however, was no bar to his having the noblest tomb in the world, at S. Lorenzo), the succession should have passed to the other branch of the Medici family, the descendants of old Giovanni's second son Lorenzo, brother of Cosimo. But Giulio, at Rome, always at the ear of the indolent, pleasure-loving Leo X, had other projects. Born in 1478, the illegitimate son of a charming father, Giulio had none of the great Medici traditions, and the Medici name never stood so low as during his period of power. Himself illegitimate, he was the father of an illegitimate son, Alessandro, for whose advancement he toiled much as Alexander VI had toiled for that of Caesar Borgia. He had not the black, bold wickedness of Alexander VI, but as Pope Clement VII, which he became in 1523, he was little less admirable. He was cunning, ambitious, and tyrannical, and during his pontificate he contrived not only to make many powerful enemies and to see both Rome and Florence under siege, but to lose England for the Church.

We move, however, too fast. The year is 1519 and Lorenzo is dead, and the rightful heir to the Medici wealth and power was to be kept out. To do this Giulio himself moved to Florence and settled in the Medici palace, and on his return to Rome Cardinal Passerini was installed in the Medici palace in his stead, nominally as the custodian of little Catherine de' Medici and Ippolito, a boy of ten, the illegitimate son of Giuliano, Duke of Nemours. That Florence should have put up with this Roman control shows us how enfeebled was her once proud spirit. In 1521 Leo X died, to be succeeded, in spite of all Giulio's efforts, by Adrian of Utrecht, as Adrian VI, a good, sincere man who, had he lived, might have enormously changed the course not only of Italian but of English history. He survived, however, for less than two years, and then came Giulio's chance, and he was elected Pope Clement VII.

Clement's first duty was to make Florence secure, and he therefore sent his son Alessandro, then about thirteen, to join the others at the Medici palace, which thus now contained a resident cardinal, watchful of Medici interests; a legitimate daughter of Lorenzo, Duke of Urbino (but owing to quarrels she was removed to a convent); an illegitimate son of Giuliano, Duke of Nemours, the nominal heir and already a member of the Government; and the Pope's illegitimate son, of whose origin, however, nothing was said, although it was implied that Lorenzo, Duke of Nemours, was his father.

This was the state of affairs during Clement's war with the Emperor Charles V, [2] which ended with the siege of Rome and the imprisonment of the Pope in the Castle of S. Angelo for some months until he contrived to escape to Orvieto; and meanwhile Florence, realizing his powerlessness, uttered a decree again banishing the Medici family, and in 1527 they were sent forth from the city for the third time. But even now, when the move was so safe, Florence lacked courage to carry it out until a member of the Medici family, furious at the presence of the base-born Medici in the palace, and a professed hater of her base-born uncle Clement VII and all his ways–Clarice Strozzi, née Clarice de' Medici, granddaughter of Lorenzo the Magnificent–came herself to this house and drove the usurpers from it with her extremely capable tongue.

To explain clearly the position of the Florentine Republic at this time would be too deeply to delve into history, but it may briefly be said that by means of humiliating surrenders and much crafty diplomacy, Clement VII was able to bring about in 1529 peace between the Emperor Charles V and Francis I of France, by which Charles was left master of Italy, while his partner and ally in these transactions, Clement, expected for his own share certain benefits in which the humiliation of Florence and the exaltation of Alessandro came first. Florence, having taken sides with Francis, found herself in any case very badly left, with the result that at the end of 1529 Charles V's army, with the papal forces to assist, laid siege to her. The siege lasted for ten months, in which the city was most ably defended by Ferrucci, that gallant soldier whose portrait by Piero di Cosimo is in our National Gallery–No. 895–and then came a decisive battle in which the Emperor and Pope were conquerors, a thousand brave Florentines were put to death and others were imprisoned.

Alessandro de' Medici arrived at the Medici palace in 1531, and in 1532 the glorious Florentine Republic of so many years' growth, for the establishment of which so much good blood had been spilt, was declared to be at an end. Alessandro being proclaimed Duke, his first act was to order the demolition of the great bell of the Signoria which had so often called the citizens to arms or meetings of independence.

Meanwhile Ippolito, the natural son of Giuliano, Duke of Nemours, and therefore the rightful heir, after having been sent on various missions by Clement VII, to keep him out of the way, settled at Bologna and took to poetry. He was a kindly, melancholy man with a deep sense of human injustice;

and in 1535, when, after Clement VII's very welcome demise, the Florentine exiles who either had been banished from Florence by Alessandro or had left of their own volition rather than live in the city under such a contemptible ruler, sent an embassy to the Emperor Charles V to help them against this new tyrant, Ippolito headed it; but Alessandro prudently arranged for his assassination en route.

It is unlikely, however, that the Emperor would have done anything, for in the following year he allowed his daughter Margaret to become Alessandro's wife. That was in 1536. In January, 1537, Lorenzino de' Medici, a cousin, one of the younger branch of the family, assuming the mantle of Brutus, or liberator, stabbed Alessandro to death while he was keeping an assignation in the house that then adjoined this palace. Thus died, at the age of twenty-six, one of the most worthless of men, and, although illegitimate, the last of the direct line of Cosimo de' Medici, the Father of his Country, to govern Florence.

The next ruler came from the younger branch, to which we now turn. Old Giovanni di Bicci had two sons, Cosimo and Lorenzo. Lorenzo's son, Pier Francesco de' Medici, had a son Giovanni de' Medici. This Giovanni, who married Caterina Sforza of Milan, had also a son named Giovanni, born in 1498, and it was he who was the rightful heir when Lorenzo, Duke of Urbino, died in 1519. He was connected with both sides of the family, for his father, as I have said, was the great grandson of the first Medici on our list, and his wife was Maria Salviati, daughter of Lucrezia de' Medici–herself a daughter of Lorenzo the Magnificent–and Jacopo Salviati, a wealthy Florentine. When, however, Lorenzo, Duke of Urbino, died in 1519, Giovanni was a young man of twenty-one with an absorbing passion for fighting, which Clement VII (then Giulio) was only too keen to foster, since he wished him out of the way in order that his own projects for the ultimate advancement of the base-born Alessandro, and meanwhile of the catspaw, the base-born Ippolito, might be furthered. Giovanni had already done some good service in the field, was becoming famous as the head of his company of Black

Bands, and was known as Giovanni delle Bande Nere; and his marriage to his cousin Maria Salviati and the birth of his only son Cosimo in 1519 made no difference to his delight in warfare. He was happy only when in the field of battle, and the struggle between Francis and Charles gave him ample opportunities, fighting on the side of Charles and the Pope and doing many brave and dashing things. He died at an early age, only twenty-eight, in 1526, the idol of his men, leaving a widow and child in poverty.

Almost immediately afterwards came the third banishment of the Medici family from Florence. Giovanni's widow and their son Cosimo got along as best they could until the murder of Alessandro in 1537, when Cosimo was nearly eighteen. He was a quiet, reserved youth, who had apparently taken but little interest in public affairs, and had spent his time in the country with his mother, chiefly in field sports. But no sooner was Alessandro dead, and his slayer Lorenzino had escaped, than Cosimo approached the Florentine council and claimed to be appointed to his rightful place as head of the State, and this claim he put, or suggested, with so much humility that his wish was granted. Instantly one of the most remarkable transitions in history occurred: the youth grew up almost in a day and at once began to exert unsuspected reserves of power and authority. In despair a number of the chief Florentines made an effort to depose him, and a battle was fought at Montemurlo, a few miles from Florence, between Cosimo's troops, fortified by some French allies, and the insurgents. That was in 1537; the victory fell to Cosimo; and his long and remarkable reign began with the imprisonment and execution of the chief rebels.

Although Cosimo made so bloody a beginning he was the first imaginative and thoughtful administrator that Florence had had since Lorenzo the Magnificent. He set himself grimly to build upon the ruins which the past forty and more years had produced; and by the end of his reign he had worked wonders. As first he lived in the Medici palace, but after marrying a wealthy wife, Eleanora of Toledo, he transferred his home to the Signoria, now called the Palazzo Vecchio, as a safer spot, and established a bodyguard of Swiss lancers in Orcagna's loggia, close by. [3] Later he bought the unfinished Pitti palace with his wife's money, finished it, and moved there. Meanwhile he was strengthening his position in every way by alliances and treaties, and also by the convenient murder of Lorenzino, the Brutus who had rid Florence of Alessandro ten years earlier, and whose presence in the flesh could not but be a cause of anxiety since Lorenzino derived from an elder son of the Medici, and Cosimo from a younger. In 1555 the ancient republic of Siena fell to Cosimo's troops after a cruel and barbarous siege and was thereafter merged in Tuscany, and in 1570 Cosimo assumed the title of Cosimo I, Grand Duke of Tuscany, and was crowned at Rome.

Whether or not the common accusation against the Medici as a family, that they had but one motive–mercenary ambition and self-aggrandisement–is true, the fact remains that the crown did not reach their brows until one hundred and seventy years from the first appearance of old Giovanni di Bicci in Florentine affairs. The statue of Cosimo I in the Piazza della Signoria has a bas-relief of his coronation. He was then fifty-one; he lived but four more years, and when he died he left a dukedom flourishing in every way: rich, powerful, busy, and enlightened. He had developed and encouraged the arts, capriciously, as Cellini's "Autobiography" tells us, but genuinely too, as we can see at the Uffizi and the Pitti. The arts, however, were not what they had been, for the great period had passed and Florence was in the trough of the wave. Yet Cosimo found the best men he could–Cellini, Bronzino, and Vasari–and kept them busy. But his greatest achievement as a connoisseur was his interest in Etruscan remains and the excavations at Arezzo and elsewhere which yielded the priceless relics now at the Archaeological Museum.

With Cosimo I this swift review of the Medici family ends. The rest have little interest for the visitor to Florence to-day, for whom Cellini's Perseus, made to Cosimo I's order, is the last great artistic achievement in the city in point of time. But I may say that Cosimo I's direct descendants occupied the throne (as it had now become) until the death of Gian Gastone, son of Cosimo III, who died in 1737. Tuscany passed to Austria until 1801. In 1807 it became French, and in 1814 Austrian again. In 1860 it was merged in the Kingdom of Italy under the rule of the monarch who has given his name to the great new Piazza–Vittorio Emmanuele.

After Gian Gastone's death one other Medici remained alive: Anna Maria Ludovica, daughter of Cosimo III. Born in 1667, she married the Elector Palatine of the Rhine, and survived until 1743. It was she who left to the city the priceless Medici collections, as I have stated in chapter VIII. The earlier and greatest of the Medici are buried in the church of S. Lorenzo or in Michelangelo's sacristy; the later Medici, beginning with Giovanni delle Bande Nere and his wife, and their son Cosimo I, are in the gorgeous mausoleum that adjoins S. Lorenzo and is still being enriched with precious marbles.

Such is an outline of the history of this wonderful family, and we leave their ancient home, built by the greatest and wisest of them, with mixed feelings of admiration and pity. They were seldom lovable; they were often despicable; but where they were great they were very great indeed. A Latin inscription in the courtyard reminds the traveller of the distinction which the house possesses, calling it the home not only of princes but of knowledge herself and a treasury of the arts. But Florence, although it bought the palace from the Riccardi family a century and more ago, has never cared to give it back its rightful name.

CHAPTER VI

. Lorenzo and Michelangelo

S
A forlorn façade–The church of the Medici–Cosimo's parents' tomb–Donatello's cantoria and pulpits–Brunelleschi's sacristy–Donatello again–The palace of the dead Grand Dukes–Costly intarsia–Michelangelo's sacristy–A weary Titan's life–The victim of capricious pontiffs–The Medici tombs–Mementi mori–The Casa Buonarroti–Brunelleschi's cloisters–A model library.

Architecturally S. Lorenzo does not attract as S. Croce and S. Maria Novella do; but certain treasures of sculpture make it unique. Yet it is a cool scene of noble grey arches, and the ceiling is very happily picked out with gold and colour. Savonarola preached some of his most important sermons here; here Lorenzo the Magnificent was married.

The façade has never yet been finished: it is just ragged brickwork waiting for its marble, and likely to wait, although such expenditure on marble is going on within a few yards of it as makes one gasp. Not very far away, in the Via Ghibellina, is a house which contains some rough plans by a master hand for this façade, drawn some four hundred years ago–the hand of none other than Michelangelo, whose scheme was to make it not only a wonder of architecture but a wonder also of statuary, the façade having many niches, each to be filled with a sacred figure. But Michelangelo always dreamed on a scale utterly disproportionate to the foolish little span of life allotted to us and the S. Lorenzo façade was never even begun.

The piazza which these untidy bricks overlook is now given up to stalls and is the centre of the cheap clothing district. Looking diagonally across it from the church one sees the great walls of the courtyard of what is now the Riccardi palace, but was in the great days the Medici palace; and at the corner, facing the Borgo S. Lorenzo, is Giovanni delle Bande Nere, in stone, by the impossible Bandinelli, looking at least twenty years older than he ever lived to be.

S. Lorenzo was a very old church in the time of Giovanni de' Medici, the first great man of the family, and had already been restored once, in the eleventh century, but it was his favourite church, chosen by him for his own resting-place, and he spent great sums in improving it. All this with the assistance of Brunelleschi, who is responsible for the interior as we now see it, and would, had he lived, have completed the façade. After Giovanni came Cosimo, who also devoted great sums to the glory of this church, not only assisting Brunelleschi with his work but inducing Donatello to lavish his genius upon it; and the church was thus established as the family vault of the Medici race. Giovanni lies here; Cosimo lies here; and Piero; while Lorenzo the Magnificent and Giuliano and certain descendants were buried in the Michelangelo sacristy, and all the Grand Dukes in the ostentatious chapel behind the altar.

Cosimo is buried beneath the floor in front of the high altar, in obedience to his wish, and by the special permission of the Roman Church; and in the same vault lies Donatello. Cosimo, who was buried with all simplicity on August 22nd, 1464, in his last illness recommended Donatello, who was then seventy-eight, to his son Piero. The old sculptor survived his illustrious patron and friend only two and a half years, declining gently into the grave, and his body was brought here in December, 1466. A monument to his memory was erected in the church in 1896. Piero (the Gouty), who survived until 1469, lies close by, his bronze monument, with that of his brother, being that between the sacristy and the adjoining chapel, in an imposing porphyry and bronze casket, the work of Verrocchio, one of the richest and most impressive of all the memorial sculptures of the Renaissance. The marble pediment is supported by four tortoises, such as support the monoliths in the Piazza S. Maria Novella. The iron rope work that divides the sacristy from the chapel is a marvel of workmanship.

But we go too fast: the church before the sacristy, and the glories of the church are Donatello's. We have seen his cantoria in the Museum of the Cathedral. Here is another, not so riotous and jocund in spirit, but in its own way hardly less satisfying. The Museum cantoria has the wonderful frieze of dancing figures; this is an exercise in marble intarsia. It has the same row of pillars with little specks of mosaic gold; but its beauty is that of delicate proportions and soft tones. The cantoria is in the left aisle, in its original place; the two bronze pulpits are in the nave. These have a double interest as being not only Donatello's work but his latest work. They were incomplete at his death, and were finished by his pupil Bertoldo (1410-1491), and since, as we shall see, Bertoldo became the master of Michelangelo, when he was a lad of fifteen and Bertoldo an old man of eighty, these pulpits may be said to form a link between the two great S. Lorenzo sculptors. How fine and free and spirited Bertoldo could be, alone, we shall see at the Bargello. The S. Lorenzo pulpits are very difficult to study: nothing wants a stronger light than a bronze relief, and in Florence students of bronze reliefs are accustomed to it, since the most famous of all–the Ghiberti doors–are in the open air. Only in course of time can one discern the scenes here. The left pulpit is the finer, for it contains the "Crucifixion" and the "Deposition," which to me form the most striking of the panels.

The other piece of sculpture in the church itself is a ciborium by Desiderio da Settignano, in the chapel at the end of the right transept–an exquisite work by this rare and playful and distinguished hand. It is fitting that Desiderio should be here, for he was Donatello's favourite pupil. The S. Lorenzo ciborium is wholly charming, although there is a "Deposition" upon it; the little Boy is adorable; but one sees it with the greatest difficulty owing to the crowded state of the altar and the dim light. The altar picture in the Martelli chapel, where the sympathetic Donatello monument (in the same medium as his "Annunciation" at S. Croce) is found–on the way to the Library–is by Lippo Lippi, and is notable for the pretty Virgin receiving the angel's news. There is nice colour in the predella.

As I have said in the first chapter, we are too prone to ignore the architect. We look at the jewels and forget the casket. Brunelleschi is a far greater maker of Florence than either Donatello or Michelangelo; but one thinks of him rather as an abstraction than a man or forgets him altogether. Yet the S. Lorenzo sacristy is one of the few perfect things in the world. What most people, however, remember is its tombs, its doors, and its reliefs; the proportions escape them. I think its shallow easy dome beyond description beautiful. Brunelleschi, who had an investigating genius, himself painted the quaint constellations in the ceiling over the altar. At the Pazzi chapel we shall find similar architecture; but there extraneous colour was allowed to come in. Here such reliefs as were admitted are white too.

The tomb under the great marble and porphyry table in the centre is that of Giovanni di Bicci, the father, and Piccarda, the mother, of Cosimo Pater, and is usually attributed to Buggiano, the adopted son of Brunelleschi, but other authorities give it either to Donatello alone or to Donatello with Michelozzo: both from the evidence of the design and because it is unlikely that Cosimo would ask any one else than one of these two friends of his to carry out a commission so near his heart. The table is part of the scheme and not a chance covering. I think the porphyry centre ought to be movable, so that the beautiful flying figures on the sarcophagus could be seen. But Donatello's most striking achievement here is the bronze doors, which are at once so simple and so strong and so surprising by the activity of the virile and spirited holy men, all converting each other, thereon depicted. These doors could not well be more different from Ghiberti's, in the casting of which Donatello assisted; those in such high relief, these so low; those so fluid and placid, and these so vigorous.

Donatello presides over this room (under Brunelleschi). The vivacious, speaking terra-cotta bust of the young S. Lorenzo on the altar is his; the altar railing is probably his; the frieze of terra-cotta cherubs may be his; the four low reliefs in the spandrels, which it is so difficult to discern but which photographs prove to be wonderful scenes in the life of S. John the Evangelist–so like, as one peers up at them, plastic Piranesis, with their fine masonry–are his. The other reliefs are Donatello's too; but the lavabo in the inner sacristy is Verrocchio's, and Verrocchio's tomb of Piero can never be overlooked even amid such a wealth of the greater master's work.

From this fascinating room–fascinating both in itself and in its possessions–we pass, after distributing the necessary largesse to the sacristan, to a turnstile which admits, on payment of a lira, to the Chapel of the Princes and to Michelangelo's sacristy. Here is contrast, indeed: the sacristy, austere and classic, and the chapel a very exhibition building of floridity and coloured ornateness, dating from the seventeenth century and not finished yet. In paying the necessary fee to see these buildings one thinks again what the feelings of Giovanni and Cosimo and Lorenzo the Magnificent, and even of Cosimo I, all such generous patrons of Florence, would be, if they could see the present feverish collection of lire in their beautiful city.

Of the Chapel of the Princes I have little to say. To pass from Michelangelo's sacristy to this is an error; see it, if see it you must, first. While the façade of S. Lorenzo is still neglected and the cornice of Brunelleschi's dome is still unfinished, this lapidary's show-room is being completed at a cost of millions of lire. Ever since 1888 has the floor been in progress, and there are many years' work yet. An enthusiastic custodian gave me a list of the stones which were used in the designs of the coats of arms of Tuscan cities, of which that of Fiesole is the most attractive:–Sicily jasper, French jasper, Tuscany jasper, petrified wood, white and yellow, Corsican granite, Corsican jasper, Oriental alabaster, French marble, lapis lazuli, verde antico, African marble, Siena marble, Carrara marble, rose agate, mother of pearl, and coral. The names of the Medici are in porphyry and ivory. It is all very marvellous and occasionally beautiful; but...

This pretentious building was designed by a natural son of Cosimo I in 1604, and was begun as the state mausoleum of the Grand Dukes; and all lie here. All the Grand Duchesses too, save Bianca Capella, wife of Francis I, who was buried none knows where. It is strange to realize as one stands here that this pavement covers all those ladies, buried in their wonderful clothes. We shall see Eleanor of Toledo, wife of Cosimo I, in Bronzino's famous picture at the Uffizi, in an amazing brocaded dress: it is that dress in which she reposes beneath us! They had their jewels too, and each Grand Duke his crown and sceptre; but these, with one or two exceptions, were stolen during the French occupation of Tuscany, 1801-1814. Only two of the Grand Dukes have their statues–Ferdinand I and Cosimo II–and the Medici no longer exist in the Florentine memory; and yet the quiet brick floor is having all this money squandered on it to superimpose costly marbles which cannot matter to anybody.

Michelangelo's chapel, called the New Sacristy, was begun for Leo X and finished for Giulio de' Medici, illegitimate son of the murdered Giuliano and afterwards Pope Clement VII. Brunelleschi's design for the Old Sacristy was followed but made more severe. This, one would feel to be the very home of dead princes even if there were no statues. The only colours are the white of the walls and the brown of the pillars and windows; the dome was to have been painted, but it fortunately escaped.

The contrast between Michelangelo's dome and Brunelleschi's is complete–Brunelleschi's so suave and gentle in its rise, with its grey lines to help the eye, and this soaring so boldly to its lantern, with its rigid device of dwindling squares. The odd thing is that with these two domes to teach him better the designer of the Chapel of the Princes should have indulged in such floridity.

Such is the force of the architecture in the sacristy that one is profoundly conscious of being in melancholy's most perfect home; and the building is so much a part of Michelangelo's life and it contains such marvels from his hand that I choose it as a place to tell his story. Michelangelo Buonarroti was born on March 6th, 1475, at Caprese, of which town his father was Podestà. At that time Brunelleschi had been dead twenty-nine years, Fra Angelico twenty years, Donatello nine years, Leonardo da Vinci was twenty-three years old, and Raphael was not yet born. Lorenzo the Magnificent had been on what was virtually the throne of Florence since 1469 and was a young man of twenty-six. For foster-mother the child had the wife of a stone-mason at Settignano, whither the family soon moved, and Michelangelo used to say that it was with her milk that he imbibed the stone-cutting art. It was from the air too, for Settignano's principal industry was sculpture. The village being only three miles from Florence, from it the boy could see the city very much as we see it now–its Duomo, its campanile, with the same attendant spires. He was sent to Florence to school and intended for either the wool or silk trade, as so many Florentines were; but displaying artistic ability, he induced his father to apprentice him, at the age of thirteen, to a famous goldsmith and painter of Florence who had a busy atelier–no other than Domenico Ghirlandaio, who was then a man of thirty-nine.

Michelangelo remained with him for three years, and although his power and imagination were already greater than his master's, he learned much, and would never have made his Sixtine Chapel frescoes with the ease he did but for this early grounding. For Ghirlandaio, although not of the first rank of painters in genius, was pre-eminently there in thoroughness, while he was good for the boy too in spirit, having a large way with him. The first work of Ghirlandaio which the boy saw in the making was the beautiful "Adoration of the Magi," in the Church of the Spedale degli Innocenti, completed in 1488, and the S. Maria Novella frescoes, and it is reasonable to suppose that he helped with the frescoes in colour grinding, even if he did not, as some have said, paint with his own hand the beggar sitting on the steps in the scene representing the "Presentation of the Virgin". That he was already clever with his pencil, we know, for he had made some caricatures and corrected a drawing or two.

The three years with Ghirlandaio were reduced eventually to one, the boy having the good fortune to be chosen as one of enough promise to be worth instruction, both by precept and example, in the famous Medici garden. Here he was more at home than in a painting room, for plastic art was his passion, and not only had Lorenzo the Magnificent gathered together there many of those masterpieces of ancient sculpture which we shall see at the Uffizi, but Bertoldo, the aged head of this informal school, was the possessor of a private collection of Donatellos and other Renaissance work of extraordinary beauty and worth. Donatello's influence on the boy held long enough for him to make the low relief of the Madonna, much in his style, which is now preserved in the Casa Buonarroti, while the plaque of the battle of the Centaurs and Lapithae which is also there shows Bertoldo's influence.

The boy's first encounter with Lorenzo occurred while he was modelling the head of an aged faun. His magnificent patron stopped to watch him, pointing out that so old a creature would probably not have such a fine set of teeth, and Michelangelo, taking the hint, in a moment had not only knocked out a tooth or two but–and here his observation told–hollowed the gums and cheeks a little in sympathy. Lorenzo was so pleased with his quickness and skill that he received him into his house as the companion of his three sons: of Piero, who was so soon and so disastrously to succeed his father, but was now a high-spirited youth; of Giovanni, who, as Pope Leo X many years after, was to give Michelangelo the commission for this very sacristy; and of Giuliano, who lies beneath one of the tombs. As their companion he enjoyed the advantage of sharing their lessons under Poliziano, the poet, and of hearing the conversation of Pico della Mirandola, who was usually with Lorenzo; and to these early fastidious and intellectual surroundings the artist owed much.

That he read much, we know, the Bible and Dante being constant companions; and we know also that in addition to modelling and copying under Bertoldo, he was assiduous in studying Masaccio's frescoes at the church of the Carmine across the river, which had become a school of painting. It was there that his fellow-pupil, Pietro Torrigiano, who was always his enemy and a bully, broke his nose with one blow and flew to Rome from the rage of Lorenzo.

It was when Michelangelo was seventeen that Lorenzo died, at the early age of forty-two, and although the garden still existed and the Medici palace was still open to the youth, the spirit had passed. Piero, who succeeded his father, had none of his ability or sagacity, and in two years was a refugee from the city, while the treasures of the garden were disposed by auction, and Michelangelo, too conspicuous as a Medici protégé to be safe, hurried away to Bologna. He was now nineteen.

Of his travels I say nothing here, for we must keep to Florence, whither he thought it safe to return in 1495. The city was now governed by the Great Council and the Medici banished. Michelangelo remained only a brief time and then went to Rome, where he made his first Pietà, at which he was working during the trial and execution of Savonarola, whom he admired and reverenced, and where he remained until 1501, when, aged twenty-six, he returned to Florence to do some of his most famous work. The Medici were still in exile.

It was in August, 1501, that the authorities of the cathedral asked Michelangelo to do what he could with a great block of marble on their hands, from which he carved that statue of David of which I tell the story in chapter XVI. This established his pre-eminence as a sculptor. Other commissions for statues poured in, and in 1504 he was invited to design a cartoon for the Palazzo Vecchio, to accompany one by Leonardo, and a studio was given him in the Via Guelfa for the purpose. This cartoon, when finished, so far established him also as the greatest of painters that the Masaccios in the Carmine were deserted by young artists in order that this might be studied instead. The cartoon, as I relate in the chapter on the Palazzo Vecchio, no longer exists.

The next year, 1505, Michelangelo, nearing his thirtieth birthday, returned to Rome and entered upon the second and tragic period of his life, for he arrived there only to receive the order for the Julius tomb which poisoned his remaining years, and of which more is said in the chapter on the Accademia, where we see so many vestiges of it both in marble and plaster. But I might remark here that this vain and capricious pontiff, whose pride and indecision robbed the world of no one can ever say what glorious work from Michelangelo's hand, is the benevolent-looking old man whose portrait by Raphael is in the Pitti and Uffizi in colour, in the Corsini Palace in charcoal, and again in our own National Gallery in colour.

Of Michelangelo at Rome and Carrara, whither he went to superintend in person the quarrying of the marble that was to be transferred to life and where he had endless vexations and mortifications, I say nothing. Enough that the election of his boy friend Giovanni de' Medici as Pope Leo X in 1513 brought him again to Florence, the Pope having a strong wish that Michelangelo should complete the façade of the Medici family church, S. Lorenzo, where we now are. As we know, the scheme was not carried out, but in 1520 the Pope substituted another and more attractive one: namely, a chapel to contain the tombs not only of his father the Magnificent, and his uncle, who had been murdered in the Duomo many years before, but also his nephew Piero de' Medici, Duke of Urbino, who had just died, in 1519, and his younger brother (and Michelangelo's early playmate) Giuliano de' Medici, Duke of Nemours, who had died in 1516. These were not Medici of the highest class, but family pride was strong. It is, however, odd that no memorial of Piero di Lorenzo de' Medici, who had been drowned at the age of twenty-two in 1503, was required; perhaps it may have been that since it was Piero's folly that had brought the Medici into such disgrace in 1494, the less thought of him the better.

Michelangelo took fire at once, and again hastened to Carrara to arrange for marble to be sent to his studio in the Via Mozzi, now the Via S. Zenobi; while the building stone was brought from Fiesole. Leo X lived only to know that the great man had begun, the new patron being Giulio de' Medici, natural son of the murdered Giuliano, now a cardinal, and soon, in 1523, to become Pope Clement VII. This Pope showed deep interest in the project, but wished not only to add tombs of himself and Pope Leo X, but also to build a library for the Laurentian collection, which Michelangelo must design. A little later he had decided that he would prefer to lie in the choir of the church, and Leo X with him, and instead therefore of tombs Michelangelo might merely make a colossal statue of him to stand in the piazza before the church. The sculptor's temper had not been improved by his many years' experience of papal caprice, and he replied to this suggestion with a letter unique even in the annals of infuriated artists. Let the statue be made, of course, he said, but let it be useful as well as ornamental: the lower portion to be also a barber's shop, and the head, since it would be empty, a greengrocer's. The Pope allowed himself to be rebuked, and abandoned the statue, writing a mild and even pathetic reply.

Until 1527 Michelangelo worked away at the building and the tombs, always secretly, behind impenetrable barriers; and then came the troubles which led to the siege of Florence, following upon the banishment of Alessandro, Duke of Urbino, natural son of the very Lorenzo whom the sculptor was to dignify for all time. By the Emperor Charles V and Pope Clement VII the city was attacked, and Michelangelo was called away from Clement's sacristy to fortify Florence against Clement's soldiers. Part of his ramparts at S. Miniato still remain, and he strengthened all the gates; but, feeling himself slighted and hating the whole affair, he suddenly disappeared. One story is that he hid in the church tower of S. Niccolò, below what is now the Piazzale dedicated to his memory. Wherever he was, he was proclaimed an outlaw, and then, on Florence finding that she could not do without him, was pardoned, and so returned, the city meanwhile having surrendered and the Medici again being restored to power.

The Pope showed either fine magnanimity or compounded with facts in the interest of the sacristy; for he encouraged Michelangelo to proceed, and the pacific work was taken up once more after the martial interregnum, and in a desultory way he was busy at it, always secretly and moodily, until 1533, when he tired completely and never touched it again. A year later Clement VII died, having seen only drawings of the tombs, if those.

But though left unfinished, the sacristy is wholly satisfying–more indeed than satisfying, conquering. Whatever help Michelangelo may have had from his assistants, it is known that the symbolical figures on the tombs and the two seated Medici are from his hand. Of the two finished or practically finished tombs–to my mind as finished as they should be–that of Lorenzo is the finer. The presentment of Lorenzo in armour brooding and planning is more splendid than that of Giuliano; while the old man, whose head anticipates everything that is considered most original in Rodin's work, is among the best of Michelangelo's statuary. Much speculation has been indulged in as to the meaning of the symbolism of these tombs, and having no theory of my own to offer, I am glad to borrow Mr. Gerald S. Davies' summary from his monograph on Michelangelo. The figure of Giuliano typifies energy and leadership in repose; while the man on his tomb typifies Day and the woman Night, or the man Action and the woman the sleep and rest that produce Action. The figure of Lorenzo typifies Contemplation, the woman Dawn, and the man Twilight, the states which lie between light and darkness, action and rest. What Michelangelo–who owed nothing to any Medici save only Lorenzo the Magnificent and had seen the best years of his life frittered away in the service of them and other proud princes–may also have intended we shall never know; but he was a saturnine man with a long memory, and he might easily have made the tombs a vehicle for criticism. One would not have another touch of the chisel on either of the symbolical male figures.

Although a tomb to Lorenzo the Magnificent by Michelangelo would surely have been a wonderful thing, there is something startling and arresting in the circumstance that he has none at all from any hand, but lies here unrecorded. His grandfather, in the church itself, rests beneath a plain slab, which aimed so consciously at modesty as thereby to achieve special distinction: Lorenzo, leaving no such directions, has nothing, while in the same room are monuments to two common-place descendants to thrill the soul. The disparity is in itself monumental. That Michelangelo's Madonna and Child are on the slab which covers the dust of Lorenzo and his brother is a chance. The saints on either side are S. Cosimo and S. Damian, the patron saints of old Cosimo de' Medici, and are by Michelangelo's assistants. The Madonna was intended for the altar of the sacristy. Into this work the sculptor put much of his melancholy and, one feels, disappointment. The face of the Madonna is already sad and hopeless; but the Child is perhaps the most splendid and determined of any in all Renaissance sculpture. He may, if we like, symbolize the new generation that is always deriving sustenance from the old, without care or thought of what the old has to suffer; he crushes his head against his mother's breast in a very passion of vigorous dependence. [4]

Whatever was originally intended, it is certain that in Michelangelo's sacristy disillusionment reigns as well as death. But how beautiful it is!

In a little room leading from the sacristy I was shown by a smiling custodian Lorenzo the Magnificent's coffin, crumbling away, and photographs of the skulls of the two brothers: Giuliano's with one of Francesco de' Pazzi's dagger wounds in it, and Lorenzo's, ghastly in its decay. I gave the man half a lira.

While he was working on the tombs Michelangelo had undertaken now and then a small commission, and to this period belongs the David which we shall see in the little room on the ground floor of the Bargello. In 1534, when he finally abandoned the sacristy, and, leaving Florence for ever, settled in Rome, the Laurentian library was only begun, and he had little interest in it. He never saw it again. At Rome his time was fully occupied in painting the "Last Judgment" in the Sixtine Chapel, and in various architectural works. But Florence at any rate has two marble masterpieces that belong to the later period–the Brutus in the Bargello and the Pietà in the Duomo, which we have seen–that poignantly impressive rendering of the entombment upon which the old man was at work when he died, and which he meant for his own grave.

His death came in 1564, on February 23rd, when he was nearly eighty-nine, and his body was brought to Florence and buried amid universal grief in S. Croce, where it has a florid monument.

Since we are considering the life of Michelangelo, I might perhaps say here a few words about his house, which is only a few minutes' distant–at No. 64 Via Ghibellina–where certain early works and personal relics are preserved. Michelangelo gave the house to his nephew Leonardo; it was decorated early in the seventeenth century with scenes in the life of the master, and finally bequeathed to the city as a heritage in 1858. It is perhaps the best example of the rapacity of the Florentines; for notwithstanding that it was left freely in this way a lira is charged for admission. The house contains more collateral curiosities, as they might be called, than those in the direct line; but there are architectural drawings from the wonderful hand, colour drawings of a Madonna, a few studies, and two early pieces of sculpture–the battle of the Lapithae and Centaurs, a relief marked by tremendous vigour and full of movement, and a Madonna and Child, also in relief, with many marks of greatness upon it. In a recess in Room IV are some personal relics of the artist, which his great nephew, the poet, who was named after him, began to collect early in the seventeenth century. As a whole the house is disappointing.

Upstairs have been arranged a quantity of prints and drawings illustrating the history of Florence.

The S. Lorenzo cloisters may be entered either from a side door in the church close to the Old Sacristy or from the piazza. Although an official in uniform keeps the piazza door, they are free. Brunelleschi is again the architect, and from the loggia at the entrance to the library you see most acceptably the whole of his cathedral dome and half of Giotto's tower. It is impossible for Florentine cloisters–or indeed any cloisters–not to have a certain beauty, and these are unusually charming and light, seen both from the loggia and the ground.

Michelangelo's Biblioteca Laurenziana, which leads from them, is one of the most perfect of sombre buildings, the very home of well-ordered scholarship. The staircase is impressive, although perhaps a little too severe; the long room could not be more satisfying to the eye. Michelangelo died before it was finished, but it is his in design, even to the ceiling and cases for MSS. in which the library is so rich, and the rich red wood ceiling. Vasari, Michelangelo's pupil and friend and the biographer to whom we are so much indebted, carried on the work. His scheme of windows has been upset on the side opposite the cloisters by the recent addition of a rotunda leading from the main room. If ever rectangular windows were more exquisitely and nobly proportioned I should like to see them. The library is free for students, and the attendants are very good in calling stray visitors' attention to illuminated missals, old MSS., early books and so forth. One of Galileo's fingers, stolen from his body, used to be kept here, in a glass case, and may be here still; but I did not see it. I saw, however, the portraits, in an old volume, of Petrarch and his Laura.

This wonderful collection was begun by Cosimo de' Medici; others added to it until it became one of the most valuable in the world, not, however, without various vicissitudes incident to any Florentine institution: while one of its most cherished treasures, the Virgil of the fourth or fifth century, was even carried to Paris by Napoleon and not returned until the great year of restoration, 1816. Among the holograph MSS. is Cellini's "Autobiography". The library, in time, after being confiscated by the Republic and sold to the monks of S. Marco, again passed into the possession of a Medici, Leo X, son of Lorenzo the Magnificent, and then of Clement VII, and he it was who commissioned Michelangelo to house it with dignity.

An old daily custom in the cloisters of S. Lorenzo was the feeding of cats; but it has long since been dropped. If you look at Mr. Hewlett's "Earthwork out of Tuscany" you will find an entertaining description of what it used to be like.

CHAPTER VII

R San Michele and the Palazzo Vecchio

O

The little Bigallo–The Misericordia–Or San Michele–Andrea Orcagna–The Tabernacle–Old Glass–A company of stone saints–Donatello's S. George–Dante conferences–The Guilds of Florence–The Palazzo Vecchio–Two Towers–Bandinelli's group–The Marzocco–The Piazza della Signoria–Orcagna's Loggia–Cellini and Cosimo–The Perseus–Verrocchio's dolphin–The Great Council Hall–Leonardo da Vinci and Michelangelo's cartoons–Bandinelli's malice–The Palazzo Vecchio as a home–Two cells and the bell of independence.

Let us now proceed along the Via Calzaioli (which means street of the stocking-makers), running away from the Piazza del Duomo to the Piazza della Signoria. The fascinatingly pretty building at the corner, opposite Pisano's Baptistery doors, is the Bigallo, in the loggia of which foundling children used to be displayed in the hope that passers-by might pity them sufficiently to make them presents or even adopt them; but this custom continues no longer. The Bigallo was designed, it is thought, by Orcagna, and it is worth the minutest study.

The Company of the Bigallo, which is no longer an active force, was one of the benevolent societies of old Florence. But the greatest of these societies, still busy and merciful, is the Misericordia, whose head-quarters are just across the Via Calzaioli, in the piazza, facing the campanile, a company of Florentines pledged at a moment's notice, no matter on what they may be engaged, to assist in any charitable work of necessity. For the most part they carry ambulances to the scenes of accident and perform the last offices for the dead in the poorer districts. When on duty they wear black robes and hoods. Their headquarters comprise a chapel, with an altar by Andrea della Robbia, and a statue of the patron saint of the Misericordia, S. Sebastian. But their real patron saint is their founder, a common porter named Pietro Borsi. In the thirteenth century it was the custom for the porters and loafers connected with the old market to meet in a shelter here and pass the time away as best they could. Borsi, joining them, was distressed to find how unprofitable were the hours, and he suggested the formation of a society to be of some real use, the money to support it to be obtained by fines in payment for oaths and blasphemies. A litter or two were soon bought and the machinery started. The name was the Company of the Brothers of Mercy. That was in 1240 to 1250. To-day no Florentine is too grand to take his part, and at the head of the porter's band of brethren is the King.

Passing along the Via Calzaioli we come on the right to a noble square building with statues in its niches Or San Michele, which stands on the site of the chapel of San Michele in Orto. San Michele in Orto, or more probably in Horreo (meaning either in the garden or in the granary), was once part of a loggia used as a corn market, in which was preserved a picture by Ugolino da Siena representing the Virgin, and this picture had the power of working miracles. Early in the fourteenth century the loggia was burned down but the picture was saved (or quickly replaced), and a new building on a much larger and more splendid scale was made for it, none other than Or San Michele, the chief architect being Taddeo Gaddi, Giotto's pupil and later the constructor of the Ponte Vecchio. Where the picture then was, I cannot say–whether inside the building or out–but the principal use of the building was to serve as a granary. After 1348, when Florence was visited by that ravaging plague which Boccaccio describes in such gruesome detail at the beginning of the "Decameron" and which sent his gay company of ladies and gentlemen to the Villa Palmieri to take refuge in story telling, and when this sacred picture was more than commonly busy and efficacious, it was decided to apply the enormous sums of money given to the shrine from gratitude in beautifying the church still more, and chiefly in providing a casket worthy of holding such a pictorial treasure. Hence came about the noble edifice of to-day.

A man of universal genius was called in to execute the tabernacle: Andrea Orcagna, a pupil probably of Andrea Pisano, and also much influenced by Giotto, whom though he had not known he idolized, and one who, like Michelangelo later, was not only a painter and sculptor but an architect and a poet. Orcagna, or, to give him his right name, Andrea di Cione, for Orcagna was an abbreviation of Arcagnolo, flourished in the middle of the fourteenth century. Among his best-known works in painting are the Dantesque frescoes in the Strozzi chapel at S. Maria Novella, and that terrible allegory of Death and Judgment in the Campo Santo at Pisa, in which the gay riding party come upon the three open graves. Orcagna put all his strength into the tabernacle of Or San Michele, which is a most sumptuous, beautiful and thoughtful shrine, yet owing to the darkness of the church is almost invisible. Guides, it is true, will emerge from the gloom and hold lighted tapers to it, but a right conception of it is impossible. The famous miraculous picture over the altar is notable rather for its properties than for its intrinsic beauty; it is the panels of the altar, which contain Orcagna's most exquisite work, representing scenes in the life of the Virgin, with emblematical figures interspersed, that one wishes to see. Only the back, however, can be seen really well, and this only when a door opposite to it–in the Via Calzaioli–is opened. It should always be open, with a grille across it, that passers-by might have constant sight of this almost unknown Florentine treasure. It is in the relief of the death of the Virgin on the back that–on the extreme right–Orcagna introduced his own portrait. The marble employed is of a delicate softness, and Orcagna had enough of Giotto's tradition to make the Virgin a reality and to interest Her, for example, as a mother in the washing of Her Baby, as few painters have done, and in particular, as, according to Ruskin, poor Ghirlandaio could not do in his fresco of the birth of the Virgin Herself. It was Orcagna's habit to sign his sculpture "Andrea di Cione, painter," and his paintings "Andrea di Cione, sculptor," and thus point his versatility. By this tabernacle, by his Pisan fresco, and by the designs of the Loggia de' Lanzi and the Bigallo (which are usually given to him), he takes his place among the most interesting and various of the forerunners of the Renaissance.

Within Or San Michele you learn the secret of the stoned-up windows which one sees with regret from without. Each, or nearly each, has an altar against it. What the old glass was like one can divine from the lovely and sombre top lights in exquisite patterns that are left; that on the centre of the right wall of the church, as one enters, having jewels of green glass as lovely as any I ever saw. But blues, purples, and reds predominate.

The tabernacle apart, the main appeal of Or San Michele is the statuary and stone-work of the exterior; for here we find the early masters at their best. The building being the head-quarters of the twelve Florentine guilds, the statues and decorations were commissioned by them. It is as though our City companies should unite in beautifying the Guildhall. Donatello is the greatest artist here, and it was for the Armourers that he made his S. George, which stands now, as he carved it in marble, in the Bargello, but has a bronze substitute in its original niche, below which is a relief of the slaying of the dragon from Donatello's chisel. Of this glorious S. George more will be said later. But I may remark now that in its place here it instantly proves the modernity and realistic vigour of its sculptor. Fine though they be, all the other statues of this building are conventional; they carry on a tradition of religious sculpture such as Niccolò Pisano respected, many years earlier, when he worked at the Pisan pulpit. But Donatello's S. George is new and is as beautiful as a Greek god, with something of real human life added.

Donatello (with Michelozzo) also made the exquisite border of the niche in the Via Calzaioli façade, in which Christ and S. Thomas now stand. He was also to have made the figures (for the Merchants' Guild) but was busy elsewhere, and they fell to Verrocchio, of whom also we shall have much to see and say at the Bargello, and to my mind they are the most beautiful of all. The John the Baptist (made for the Cloth-dealers), also on this façade, is by Ghiberti of the Baptistery gates. On the façade of the Via de' Lamberti is Donatello's superb S. Mark (for the Joiners), which led to Michelangelo's criticism that he had never seen a man who looked more virtuous, and if S. Mark were really like that he would believe all his words. "Why don't you speak to me?" he also said to this statue, as Donatello had said to the Zuccone. Higher on this façade is Luca della Robbia's famous arms of the Silk-weavers, one of the perfect things. Luca also made the arms of the Guild of Merchants, with its Florentine fleur-de-lis in the midst. For the rest, Ghiberti's S. Stephen, and Ghiberti and Michelozzo's S. Matthew, on the entrance wall, are the most remarkable. The blacksmith relief is very lively and the blacksmith's saint a noble figure.

The little square reliefs let into the wall at intervals are often charming, and the stone-work of the windows is very lovely. In fact, the four walls of this fortress church are almost inexhaustible. Within, its vaulted roof is so noble, its proportions so satisfying. One should often sit quietly here, in the gloom, and do nothing.

The little building just across the way was the Guild House of the Arte della Lana, or Wool-combers, and is now the head-quarters of the Italian Dante Society, who hold a conference every Thursday in the large room over Or San Michele, gained by the flying buttress-bridge. The dark picture on the outer wall is the very Madonna to which, when its position was at the Mercato Vecchio, condemned criminals used to pray on their way to execution.

Before we leave Or San Michele and the Arte della Lana, a word on the guilds of Florence is necessary, for at a period in Florentine history between, say, the middle of the thirteenth century and the beginning of the fifteenth, they were the very powerful controllers of the domestic affairs of the city; and it is possible that it would have been better for the Florentines had they continued to be so. For Florence was essentially mercantile and the guilds were composed of business men; and it is natural that business men should know better than noblemen what a business city needed. They were divided into major guilds, chief of which were the woollen merchants–the Arte della Lana–and the silk merchants–the Calimala–and it was their pride to put their riches at the city's service. Thus, the Arte della Lana had charge of the building of the cathedral. Each of the major guilds provided a Prior, and the Priors elected the Signoria, who governed the city. It is one of the principal charges that is brought against Cosimo de' Medici that he broke the power of the guilds.

Returning to the Via Calzaioli, and turning to the right, we come very quickly to the Piazza della Signoria, and see before us, diagonally across it, the Loggia de' Lanzi and the Palazzo Vecchio, with the gleaming, gigantic figure of Michelangelo's David against the dark gateway. This, more than the Piazza del Duomo, is the centre of Florence.

The Palazzo Vecchio was for centuries called the Signoria, being the home of the Gonfalonier of Florence and the Signoria who assisted his councils. It was begun by Arnolfo, the architect of the Duomo and S. Croce, at the end of the thirteenth century, that being, as we have seen, a period of great prosperity and ambition in Florence, but many alterations and additions were made–by Michelozzo, Cronaca, Vasari, and others–to bring it to what it now is. After being the scene of many riots, executions, and much political strife and dubiety, it became a ducal palace in 1532, and is now a civic building and show-place. In the old days the Palazzo had a ringhiera, or platform, in front of it, from which proclamations were made. To know what this was like one has but to go to S. Trinità on a very fine morning and look at Ghirlandaio's fresco of the granting of the charter to S. Francis. The scene, painted in 1485, includes not only the Signoria but the Loggia de' Lanzi (then the Loggia dell' Orcagna)–both before any statues were set up.

Every façade of the Palazzo Vecchio is splendid. I cannot say which I admire more–that which one sees from the Loggia de' Lanzi, with its beautiful coping of corbels, at once so heavy and so light, with coloured escutcheons between them, or that in the Via de' Gondi, with its fine jumble of old brickwork among the stones. The Palazzo Vecchio is one of the most resolute and independent buildings in the world; and it had need to be strong, for the waves of Florentine revolt were always breaking against it. The tower rising from this square fortress has at once grace and strength and presents a complete contrast to Giotto's campanile; for Giotto's campanile is so light and delicate and reasonable and this tower of the Signoria so stern and noble. There is a difference as between a beautiful woman and a powerful man. In the functions of the two towers–the dominating towers of Florence–is a wide difference also, for the campanile calls to prayer, while for years the sombre notes of the great Signoria bell–the Vacca–rang out only to bid the citizens to conclave or battle or to sound an alarm.

It was this Vacca wich (with others) the brave Piero Capponi threatened to ring when Charles VIII wished, in 1494, to force a disgraceful treaty on the city. The scene was the Medici Palace in the Via Larga. The paper was ready for signature and Capponi would not sign. "Then I must bid my trumpets blow," said Charles. "If you sound your trumpets," Capponi replied, "we will ring our bells;" and the King gave way, for he knew that his men had no chance in this city if it rose suddenly against them.

But the glory of the Palazzo Vecchio tower–afer its proportions–is that brilliant inspiration of the architect which led him, so to speak, to begin again by setting the four columns on the top of the solid portion. These pillars are indescribably right: so solid and yet so light, so powerful and yet so comely. Their duty was to support the bells, and particularly the Vacca, when he rocked his gigantic weight of green bronze to and fro to warn the city. Seen from a distance the columns are always beautiful; seen close by they are each a tower of comfortable strength. And how the wind blows through them from the Apennines!

The David on the left of the Palazzo Vecchio main door is only a copy. The original stood there until 1873, when, after three hundred and sixty-nine years, it was moved to a covered spot in the Accademia, as we shall there see and learn its history. If we want to know what the Palazzo Vecchio looked like at the time David was placed there, a picture by Piero di Cosimo in our National Gallery tells us, for he makes it the background of his portrait of Ferrucci, No. 895.

The group on the right represents Hercules and Cacus, [5] and is by Baccio Bandinelli (1485-1560), a coarse and offensive man, jealous of most people and particularly of Michelangelo, to whom, but for his displeasing Pope Clement VII, the block of marble from which the Hercules was carved would have been given. Bandinelli in his delight at obtaining it vowed to surpass that master's David, and those who want to know what Florence thought of his effort should consult the amusing and malicious pages of Cellini's Autobiography. On its way to Bandinelli's studio the block fell into the Arrio, and it was a joke of the time that it had drowned itself to avoid its fate at the sculptor's hands. Even after he had half done it, there was a moment when Michelangelo had an opportunity of taking over the stone and turning it into a Samson, but the siege of Florence intervened, and eventually Bandinelli had his way and the hideous thing now on view was evolved.

The lion at the left end of the façade is also a copy, the original by Donatello being in the Bargello, close by; but the pedestal is Donatello's original. This lion is the Marzocco, the legendary guardian of the Florentine republic, and it stood here for four centuries and more, superseding one which was kissed as a sign of submission by thousands of Pisan prisoners in 1364. The Florentine fleur-de-lis on the pediment is very beautiful. The same lion may be seen in iron on his staff at the top of the Palazzo Vecchio tower, and again on the Bargello, bravely flourishing his lily against the sky.

The great fountain with its bronze figures at this corner is by Bartolommeo Ammanati, a pupil of Bandinelli, and the statue of Cosimo I is by Gian Bologna, who was the best of the post-Michelangelo sculptors and did much good work in Florence, as we shall see at the Bargello and in the Boboli Gardens. He studied under Michelangelo in Rome. Though born a Fleming and called a Florentine, his great fountain at Bologna, which is really a fine thing, has identified his fame with that city. Had not Ammanati's design better pleased Cosimo I, the Bologna fountain would be here, for it was designed for this piazza. Gian's best-known work is the Flying Mercury in the Bargello, which we have seen, on mantelpieces and in shop windows, everywhere; but what is considered his masterpiece is over there, in the Loggia de' Lanzi, the very beautiful building on the right of the Palazzo, the "Rape of the Sabines," a group which, to me, gives no pleasure. The bronze reliefs under the Cosimo statue–this Cosimo being, of course, far other than Cosimo de' Medici, Father of his Country: Cosimo I of Tuscany, who insisted upon a crown and reigned from 1537 to 1575–represents his assumption of rule on the death of Alessandro in 1537; his triumphant entry into Siena when he conquered it and absorbed it; and his reception of the rank of Grand Duke. Of Cosimo (whom we met in Chapter V) more will be said when we enter the Palazzo Vecchio.

Between this statue and the Loggia de' Lanzi is a bronze tablet let into the paving which tells us that it was on this very spot, in 1498, that Savonarola and two of his companions were put to death. The ancient palace on the Duomo side of the piazza is attributed in design to Raphael, who, like most of the great artists of his time, was also an architect and was the designer of the Palazzo Pandolfini in the Via San Gallo, No. 74. The Palazzo we are now admiring for its blend of massiveness and beauty is the Uguccione, and anybody who wishes may probably have a whole floor of it to-day for a few shillings a week. The building which completes the piazza on the right of us, with coats of arms on its façade, is now given to the Board of Agriculture and has been recently restored. It was once a Court of Justice. The great building at the opposite side of the piazza, where the trams start, is a good example of modern Florentine architecture based on the old: the Palazzo Landi, built in 1871 and now chiefly an insurance office. In London we have a more attractive though smaller derivative of the great days of Florentine building, in Standen's wool shop in Jermyn Street.

The Piazza della Signoria has such riches that one is in danger of neglecting some. The Palazzo Vecchio, for example, so overpowers the Loggia de' Lanzi in size as to draw the eye from that perfect structure. One should not allow this to happen; one should let the Palazzo Vecchio's solid nobility wait awhile and concentrate on the beauty of Orcagna's three arches. Coming so freshly from his tabernacle in Or San Michele we are again reminded of the versatility of the early artists.

This structure, originally called the Loggia de' Priori or Loggia d'Orcagna, was built in the fourteenth century as an open place for the delivery of proclamations and for other ceremonies, and also as a shelter from the rain, the last being a purpose it still serves. It was here that Savonarola's ordeal by fire would have had place had it not been frustrated. Vasari also gives Orcagna the four symbolical figures in the recesses in the spandrels of the arches. The Loggia, which took its new name from the Swiss lancers, or lanzi, that Cosimo I kept there–he being a fearful ruler and never comfortable without a bodyguard–is now a recognized place of siesta; and hither many people carry their poste-restante correspondence from the neighbouring post office in the Uffizi to read in comfort. A barometer and thermometer are almost the only novelties that a visitor from the sixteenth century would notice.

The statuary is both old and new; for here are genuine antiques once in Ferdinand I's Villa Medici at Rome, and such modern masterpieces as Donatello's Judith and Holofernes, Cellini's Perseus, and Gian Bologna's two muscular and restless groups. The best of the antiques is the Woman Mourning, the fourth from the end on the left, which is a superb creation.

Donatello's Judith, which gives me less pleasure than any of his work, both in the statue and in the relief, was commissioned for Cosimo de' Medici, who placed it in the courtyard or garden of the Medici palace–Judith, like David, by her brave action against a tyrant, being a champion of the Florentine republic. In 1495, after Cosimo's worthless grandson Piero de' Medici had been expelled from Florence and the Medici palace sacked, the statue was moved to the front of the Palazzo Vecchio, where the David now is, and an inscription placed on it describing it as a warning to all enemies of liberty. This position being needed for Michelangelo's David, in 1506, Judith was moved to the Loggia to the place where the Sabine group now is. In 1560 it took up its present position.

Cellini's Perseus will not quite do, I think, after Donatello and Verrocchio; but few bronzes are more famous, and certainly of none has so vivacious and exciting a story been written as Cellini's own, setting forth his disappointments, mortifications, and pride in connexion with this statue. Cellini, whatever one may think of his veracity, is a diverting and valuable writer, and the picture of Cosimo I which he draws for us is probably very near the truth. We see him haughty, familiar, capricious, vain, impulsive, clear-sighted, and easily flattered; intensely pleased to be in a position to command the services of artists and very unwilling to pay. Cellini was a blend of lackey, child, and genius. He left Francis I in order to serve Cosimo and never ceased to regret the change. The Perseus was his greatest accomplishment for Cosimo, and the narrative of its casting is terrific and not a little like Dumas. When it was uncovered in its present position all Florence flocked to the Loggia to praise it; the poets placed commendatory sonnets on the pillars, and the sculptor peacocked up and down in an ecstasy of triumph. Then, however, his troubles once more began, for Cosimo had the craft to force Cellini to name the price, and we see Cellini in an agony between desire for enough and fear lest if he named enough he would offend his patron.

The whole book is a comedy of vanity and jealousy and Florentine vigour, with Courts as a background. It is good to read it; it is good, having read it, to study once again the unfevered resolute features of Donatello's S. George.

Cellini himself we may see among the statues under the Uffizi and again in the place of honour (as a goldsmith) in the centre of the Ponte Vecchio. Looking at the Perseus and remembering Donatello, one realizes that what Cellini wanted was character. He had temperament enough but no character. Perseus is superb, commanding, distinguished, and one doesn't care a fig for it.

On entering the Palazzo Vecchio we come instantly to one of the most charming things in Florence–Verrocchio's fountain–which stands in the midst of the courtyard. This adorable work–a little bronze Cupid struggling with a spouting dolphin–was made for Lorenzo de' Medici's country villa at Careggi and was brought here when the palazzo was refurnished for Francis I, Cosimo I's son and successor, and his bride, Joanna of Austria, in 1565. Nothing could better illustrate the accomplishment and imaginative adaptability of the great craftsmen of the day than the two works of Verrocchio that we have now seen: the Christ and S. Thomas at Or San Michele, in Donatello and Michelozzo's niche, and this exquisite fountain splashing water so musically. Notice the rich decorations of the pillars of this courtyard and the rich colour and power of the pillars themselves. The half-obliterated frescoes of Austrian towns on the walls were made to prevent Joanna from being homesick, but were more likely, one would guess, to stimulate that malady. In the left corner is the entrance to the old armoury, now empty, with openings in the walls through which pieces might be discharged at various angles on any advancing host. The groined ceiling could support a pyramid.

The Palazzo Vecchio's ground floor is a series of thoroughfares in which people are passing continually amid huge pillars and along dark passages; but our way is up the stone steps immediately to the left on leaving the courtyard where Verrocchio's child eternally smiles, for the steps take us to that vast hall designed by Cronaca for Savonarola's Great Council, which was called into being for the government of Florence after the luckless Piero de' Medici had been banished in 1494. Here much history was made. As to its structure and its architect, Vasari, who later was called in to restore it, has a deal to say, but it is too technical for us. It was built by Simone di Pollaiuolo, who was known as Cronaca (the Chronicler) from his vivid way of telling his adventures. Cronaca (1454-1508), who was a personal friend and devotee of Savonarola, drew up his plan in consultation with Leonardo da Vinci, Michelangelo (although then so young: only nineteen or twenty) and others. Its peculiarity is that it is one of the largest rooms in existence without pillars. From the foot of the steps to the further wall I make it fifty-eight paces, and thirty wide; and the proportions strike the eye as perfect. The wall behind the steps is not at right angles with the other–and this must be as peculiar as the absence of pillars.

Once there were to be paintings here by the greatest of all, for masters no less than Leonardo and Michelangelo were commissioned to decorate it, each with a great historical painting: a high honour for the youthful Michelangelo. The loss of these works is one of the tragedies of art. Leonardo chose for his subject the battle of Anghiari, an incident of 1440 when the Florentines defeated Piccinino and saved their Republic from the Milanese and Visconti. But both the cartoon and the fresco have gone for ever, and our sense of loss is not diminished by reading in Leonardo's Thoughts on Painting the directions which he wrote for the use of artists who proposed to paint battles: one of the most interesting and exciting pieces of writing in the literature of art. Michelangelo's work, which never reached the wall of the room, as Leonardo's had done, was completed as a cartoon in 1504 to 1506 in his studio in the hospital of the dyers in Sant' Onofrio, which is now the Via Guelfa. The subject was also military: an incident in the long and bitter struggle between Florence and Pisa, when Sir John Hawkwood (then in the pay of the Pisans, before he came over finally to the Florentines) attacked a body of Florentines who were bathing in the river. The scene gave the young artist scope both for his power of delineating a spirited incident and for his drawing of the nude, and those who saw it said of this work that it was finer than anything the painter ever did. While it was in progress all the young artists came to Sant' Onofrio to study it, as they and its creator had before flocked to the Carmine, where Masaccio's frescoes had for three-quarters of a century been object-lessons to students.

What became of the cartoon is not definitely known, but Vasari's story is that Bandinelli, the sculptor of the Hercules and Cacus outside the Palazzo, who was one of the most diligent copyists of the cartoon after it was placed in a room in this building, had the key of the door counterfeited, and, obtaining entrance during a moment of tumult, destroyed the picture. The reasons given are: (1, and a very poor one) that he desired to own the pieces; (2) that he wished to deprive other and rival students of the advantage of copying it; (3) that he wanted Leonardo to be the only painter of the Palazzo to be considered; and (4, and sufficient) that he hated Michelangelo. At this time Bandinelli could not have been more than eighteen. Vasari's story is uncorroborated.

Leonardo's battle merely perished, being done in some fugitive medium; and the walls are now covered with the works of Vasari himself and his pupils and do not matter, while the ceiling is a muddle of undistinguished paint. There are many statues which also do not matter; but at the raised end is Leo X, son of Lorenzo the Magnificent, and the first Medici Pope, and at the other a colossal modern statue of Savonarola, who was in person the dominating influence here for the years between 1494 and 1497; who is to many the central figure in the history of this building; and whose last night on earth was spent with his companions in this very room. But to him we come in the chapter on S. Marco.

Many rooms in the Palazzo are to be seen only on special occasions, but the great hall is always accessible. Certain rooms upstairs, mostly with rich red and yellow floors, are also visible daily, all interesting; but most notable is the Salle de Lys, with its lovely blue walls of lilies, its glorious ceiling of gold and roses, Ghirlandaio's fresco of S. Zenobius, and the perfect marble doorway containing the wooden doors of Giuliano and Benedetto da Maiano, with the heads of Dante and Petrarch in intarsia. Note the figures of Charity and Temperance in the doorway and the charming youthful Baptist.

In Eleanor of Toledo's dining-room there are some rich and elaborate green jugs which I remember very clearly and also the ceiling of her workroom with its choice of Penelope as the presiding genius. Both Eleanor's chapel and that in which Savonarola prayed before his execution are shown.

But the most popular room of all with visitors–and quite naturally–is the little boudoiresque study of Francis I, with its voluptuous ladies on the ceiling and the secret treasure-room leading from it, while on the way, just outside the door, is a convenient oubliette into which to push any inconvenient visitor.

The loggia, which Mr. Morley has painted from the Via Castellani, is also always accessible, and from it one has one of those pleasant views of warm roofs in which Florence abounds.

One of the most attractive of the smaller rooms usually on view is that one which leads from the lily-room and contains nothing but maps of the world: the most decorative things conceivable, next to Chinese paintings. Looking naturally for Sussex on the English map, I found Winchelsey, Battel, Rye, Lewes, Sorham, Arônde, and Cicestra.

From the map-room a little room is gained where the debates in the Great Council Hall might be secretly overheard by interested eavesdroppers, but in particular by Cosimo I. A part of the cornice has holes in it for this purppse, but on regaining the hall itself I found that the disparity in the pattern was perfectly evident even to my eye, so that every one in those suspicious days must have been aware of the listener.

The tower should certainly be ascended–not only for the view and to be so near the bells and the pillars, but also for historic associations. After a little way we come to the cell where Cosimo de' Medici, later to be the Father of his Country, was imprisoned, before that exile which ended in recall and triumph in 1433. This cell, although not exactly "a home from home," is possible. What is to be said of that other, some thousands of steps (as it seems) higher, where Savonarola was kept for forty days, varied only by intervals of torture? For Savonarola's cell, which is very near the top, is nothing but a recess in the wall with a door to it. It cannot be more than five feet wide and eight feet long, with an open loophole to the wind. If a man were here for forty days and then pardoned his life would be worth very little. A bitter eyrie from which to watch the city one had risked all to reform. What thoughts must have been his in that trap! What reviews of policy! What illuminations as to Florentine character!

CHAPTER VIII

THE Uffizi I: The Building and the Collectors

The growth of a gallery–Vasari's Passaggio–Cosimo I–Francis I–Ferdinand I–Ferdinand II–Cosimo III–Anna Maria Ludovica de' Medici–Pietro-Leopoldo–The statues of the façade–Art, literature, arms, science, and learning–The omissions–Florentine rapacity–An antique custom–Window views–The Uffizi drawings–The best picture.

The foreigner should understand at once that any inquiries into the history of the Uffizi family–such as for example yield interesting results in the case of the Pazzi and the Albizzi–are doomed to failure; because Uffizi merely means offices. The Palazzo degli Uffizi, or palace of offices, was built by Vasari, the biographer of the artists, for Cosimo I, who having taken the Signoria, or Palazzo Vecchio, for his own home, wished to provide another building for the municipal government. It was begun in 1560 and still so far fulfils its original purpose as to contain the general post office, while it also houses certain Tuscan archives and the national library.

A glance at Piero di Cosimo's portrait of Ferrucci in our National Gallery will show that an ordinary Florentine street preceded the erection of the Uffizi.

At that time the top storey of the building, as it now exists, was an open terrace affording a pleasant promenade from the Palazzo Vecchio down to the river and back to the Loggia de' Lanzi. Beneath this were studios and workrooms where Cosimo's army of artists and craftsmen (with Bronzino and Cellini as the most famous) were kept busy; while the public offices were on the ground floor. Then, as his family increased, Cosimo decided to move, and the incomplete and abandoned Pitti Palace was bought and finished. In 1565, as we have seen, Francis, Cosimo's son, married and was installed in the Palazzo Vecchio, and it was then that Vasari was called upon to construct the Passaggio which unites the Palazzo Vecchio and the Pitti, crossing the river by the Ponte Vecchio–Cosimo's idea (borrowed it is said from Homer's description of the passage uniting the palaces of Priam and Hector) being not only that he and his son might have access to each other, but that in the event of danger on the other side of the river a body of soldiers could be swiftly and secretly mobilized there.

Cosimo I died in 1574, and Francis I (1574-1587) succeeded him not only in rule but in that patronage of the arts which was one of the finest Medicean traditions; and it was he who first thought of making the Uffizi a picture gallery. To do this was simple: it merely meant the loss of part of the terrace by walling and roofing it in. Ferdinand I (1587-1609) added the pretty Tribuna and other rooms, and brought hither a number of the treasures from the Villa Medici at Rome. Cosimo II (1609-1621) did little, but Ferdinand II (1621-1670) completed the roofing in of the terraces, placed there his own collection of drawings and a valuable collection of Venetian pictures which he had bought, together with those that his wife Vittoria della Rovere had brought him from Urbino, while his brothers, Cardinal Giovanni Carlo de' Medici and Cardinal Leopoldo de' Medici (the extremely ugly man with the curling chin, at the head of the Uffizi stairs), added theirs. Giovanni Carlo's pictures, which mostly went to the Pitti were varied; but Leopold's were chiefly portraits of artists, wherever possible painted by themselves, a collection which is steadily being added to at the present time and is to be seen in several rooms of the Uffizi, and those miniature portraits of men of eminence which we shall see in the corridor between the Poccetti Gallery and Salon of Justice at the Pitti. Cosimo III (1670-1723) added the Dutch pictures and the famous Venus de' Medici and other Tribuna statuary.

The galleries remained the private property of the Medici family until the Electress Palatine, Anna Maria Ludovica de' Medici, daughter of Cosimo III and great niece of the Cardinal Leopold, bequeathed all these treasures, to which she had greatly added, together with bronzes now in the Bargello, Etruscan antiquities now in the Archaeological Museum, tapestries also there, and books in the Laurentian library, to Florence for ever, on condition that they should never be removed from Florence and should exist for the benefit of the public. Her death was in 1743, and with her passed away the last descendant of that Giovanni de' Medici (1360-1429) whom we saw giving commissions to Donatello, building the children's hospital, and helping Florence to the best of his power: so that the first Medici and the last were akin in love of art and in generosity to their beautiful city.

The new Austrian Grand Dukes continued to add to the Uffizi, particularly Pietro-Leopoldo (1765-1790), who also founded the Accademia. To him was due the assembling, under the Uffizi roof, of all the outlying pictures then belonging to the State, including those in the gallery of the hospital of S. Maria Nuova, which owned, among others, the famous Hugo van der Goes. It was he also who brought together from Rome the Niobe statues and constructed a room for them. Leopold II added the Iscrizioni.

It was as recently as 1842 to 1856 that the statues of the great Florentines were placed in the portico. These, beginning at the Palazzo Vecchio, are, first, against the inner wall, Cosimo Pater (1389-1464) and Lorenzo the Magnificent (1450-1492); then, outside: Orcagna; Andrea Pisano, of the first Baptistery doors; Giotto and Donatello; Alberti, who could do everything and who designed the façade of S. Maria Novella; Leonardo and Michelangelo. Next, three poets, Dante (1265-1321), Francesco Petrarca (1304-1374), and Giovanni Boccaccio (1313-1375). Then Niccolò Machiavelli (1469-1527), the statesman, and Francesco Guicciardini (1482-1540), the historian. That completes the first side.

At the end are Amerigo Vespucci (1451-1516), the explorer, who gave his name to America, and Galileo Galilei (1564-1642), the astronomer; and above is Cosimo I, the first Grand Duke.

On the Uffizi's river façade are four figures only–and hundreds of swallows' nests. The figures are Francesco Ferrucci, who died in 1530, the general painted by Piero di Cosimo in our National Gallery, who recaptured Volterra from Pope Clement VII in 1529; Giovanni delle Bande Nere (1500-1527), father of Cosimo I, and a great fighting man; Piero Capponi, who died in 1496, and delivered Florence from Charles VIII in 1494, by threatening to ring the city bells; and Farinata degli Uberti, an earlier soldier, who died in 1264 and is in the "Divina Commedia" as a hero. It was he who repulsed the Ghibelline suggestion that Florence should be destroyed and the inhabitants emigrate to Empoli.

Working back towards the Loggia de' Lanzi we find less-known names: Pietro Antonio Michele (1679-1737), the botanist; Francesco Redi (1626-1697), a poet and a man of science; Paolo Mascagni (1732-1815), the anatomist; Andrea Cesalpino (1519-1603), the philosopher; S. Antonio (died 1461), Prior of the Convent of S. Marco and Archbishop of Florence; Francesco Accorso (1182-1229), the jurist; Guido Aretino (eleventh century), musician; and Benvenuto Cellini (1500-1572), the goldsmith and sculptor. The most notable omissions are Arnolfo and Brunelleschi (but these are, as we have seen, on the façade of the Palazzo de' Canonici, opposite the south side of the cathedral), Ghiberti, Fra Angelico, and Savonarola. Personally I should like to have still others here, among them Giorgio Vasari, in recognition of his enthusiastic and entertaining biographies of the Florentine artists, to say nothing of the circumstance that he designed this building.

Before we enter any Florentine gallery let me say that there is only one free day and that the crowded Sabbath. Admittance to nearly all is a lira. Moreover, there is no re-admission. The charge strikes English visitors, accustomed to the open portals of their own museums and galleries, as an outrage, and it explains also the little interest in their treasures which most Florentines display, for being essentially a frugal people they have seldom seen them. Visitors who can satisfy the authorities that they are desirous of studying the works of art with a serious purpose can obtain free passes; but only after certain preliminaries, which include a seance with a photographer to satisfy the doorkeeper, by comparing the real and counterfeit physiognomies, that no illicit transference of the precious privilege has been made. Italy is, one knows, not a rich country; but the revenue which the gallery entrance-fees represent cannot reach any great volume, and such as it is it had much better, I should say, be raised by other means. Meanwhile, the foreigner chiefly pays it. What Giovanni de' Medici and Lorenzo de' Medici, and–even more–what Anna Maria Ludovica de' Medici, who bequeathed to the State these possessions, would think could they see this feverish and implacable pursuit of pence, I have not imagination, or scorn, enough to set down.

Infirm and languid visitors should get it clearly into their heads (1) that the tour of the Uffizi means a long walk and (2) that there is a lift. You find it in the umbrella room–at every Florentine gallery and museum is an official whose one object in life is to take away your umbrella–and it costs twopence-halfpenny and is worth far more. But walking downstairs is imperative, because otherwise one would miss Silenus and Bacchus, and a beautiful urgent Mars, in bronze, together with other fine sculptured things.

One of the quaintest symbols of conservatism in Florence is the scissors of the officials who supply tickets of entrance. Apparently the perforated line is unknown in Italy; hence the ticket is divided from its counterfoil (which I assume goes to the authorities in order that they may check their horrid takings) by a huge pair of shears. These things are snip-snapping all over Italy, all day long. Having obtained your ticket you hand it to another official at a turn-stile, and at last you are free of cupidity and red tape and may breathe easily again and examine the products of the light-hearted, generous

Renaissance in the right spirit.

One should never forget, in any gallery of Florence, to look out of the windows. There is always a courtyard, a street, or a spire against the sky; and at the Uffizi there are the river and bridges and mountains. From the loggia of the Palazzo Vecchio I once saw a woman with some twenty or thirty city pigeons on the table of her little room, feeding them with maize.

Except for glimpses of the river and the Via Guicciardini which it gives, I advise no one to walk through the passage uniting the Pitti and the Uffizi–unless of course bent on catching some of the ancient thrill when armed men ran swiftly from one palace to the other to quell a disturbance or repulse an assault. Particularly does this counsel apply to wet days, when all the windows are closed and there is no air. A certain interest attaches to the myriad portraits which line the walls, chiefly of the Medici and comparatively recent worthies; but one must have a glutton's passion either for paint or history to wish to examine these. As a matter of fact, only a lightning-speed tourist could possibly think of seeing both the Uffizi and the Pitti on the same day, and therefore the need of the passage disappears. It is hard worked only on Sundays.

The drawings in the cases in the first long corridor are worth close study–covering as they do the whole range of great Italian art: from, say, Uccello to Carlo Dolci. But as they are from time to time changed it is useless to say more of them. There is also on the first landing of the staircase a room in which exhibitions of drawings of the Old Masters are held, and this is worth knowing about, not only because of the riches of the portfolios in the collection, but also because once you have passed the doors you are inside the only picture gallery in Florence for which no entrance fee is asked. How the authorities have come to overlook this additional source of revenue, I have no notion; but they have, and visitors should hasten to make the most of it for fear that a translation of these words of mine may wander into bad hands.

To name the most wonderful picture in the Uffizi would be a very difficult task. At the Accademia, if a plebiscite were taken, there is little doubt but that Botticelli's "Primavera" would win. At the Pitti I personally would name Giorgione's "Concert" without any hesitation at all; but probably the public vote would go to Raphael's "Madonna della Sedia". But the Uffizi? Here we are amid such wealth of masterpieces, and yet when one comes to pass them in review in memory none stands out as those other two I have named. Perhaps Botticelli would win again, with his "Birth of Venus". Were the Leonardo finished ... but it is only a sketch. Luca Signorelli's wild flowers in No. 74 seem to abide with me as vividly and graciously as anything; but they are but a detail and it is a very personal predilection. Perhaps the great exotic work painted far away in Belgium–the Van der Goes triptych–is the most memorable; but to choose an alien canvas is to break the rules of the game. Is it perhaps the unfinished Leonardo after all? If not, and not the Botticelli, it is beyond question that lovely adoring Madonna, so gentle and sweet, against the purest and bluest of Tuscan skies, which is attributed to Filippino Lippi: No. 1354.

CHAPTER IX

THE Uffizi II: The First Six Rooms

Lorenzo Monaco–Fra Angelico–Mariotto Albertinelli turns innkeeper–The Venetian rooms–Giorgione's death–Titian–Mantegna uniting north and south–Giovanni Bellini–Domenico Ghirlandaio–Michelangelo–Luca Signorelli–Wild flowers–Leonardo da Vinci–Paolo Uccello.

The first and second rooms are Venetian; but I am inclined to think that it is better to take the second door on the left–the first Tuscan salon–and walking straight across it come at once to the Salon of Lorenzo Monaco and the primitives. For the earliest good pictures are here. Here especially one should remember that the pictures were painted never for a gallery but for churches. Lorenzo Monaco (Lawrence the Monk, 1370-c. 1425), who gives his name to this room, was a monk of the Camaldolese order in the Monastery of the Angeli, and was a little earlier than Fra Angelico (the Angelic Brother), the more famous painting monk, whose dates are 1387-1455. Lorenzo was influenced by Taddeo Gaddi, Giotto's godson, friend, pupil, and assistant. His greatest work is this large Uffizi altar-piece–he painted nothing but altar-pieces–depicting the Coronation of the Virgin: a great gay scene of splendour, containing pretty angels who must have been the delight of children in church. The predella–and here let me advise the visitor never to overlook the predellas, where the artist often throws off formality and allows his more natural feelings to have play, almost as though he painted the picture for others and the predella for himself–is peculiarly interesting. Look, at the left, at the death of an old Saint attended by monks and nuns, whose grief is profound. One other good Lorenzo is here, an "Adoration of the Magi," No. 39, a little out of drawing but full of life.

But for most people the glory of the room is not Lorenzo the Monk, but Brother Giovanni of Fiesole, known ever more as Beato, or Fra, Angelico. Of that most adoring and most adorable of painters I say much in the chapter on the Accademia, where he is very fully represented, and it might perhaps be well to turn to those pages (227-230) and read here, on our first sight of his genius, what is said. Two Angelicos are in this room–the great triptych, opposite the chief Lorenzo, and the "Crowning of the Virgin," on an easel. The triptych is as much copied as any picture in the gallery, not, however, for its principal figures, but for the border of twelve angels round the centre panel. Angelico's benignancy and sweetness are here, but it is not the equal of the "Coronation," which is a blaze of pious fervour and glory. The group of saints on the right is very charming; but we are to be more pleased by this radiant hand when we reach the Accademia. Already, however, we have learned his love of blue. Another altar-piece with a subtle quality of its own is the early Annunciation by Simone Martini of Siena (1285-1344) and Lippo Memmi, his brother (d. 1357), in which the angel speaks his golden words across the picture through a vase of lilies, and the Virgin receives them shrinkingly. It is all very primitive, but it has great attraction, and it is interesting to think that the picture must be getting on for six hundred years of age. This Simone was a pupil of Giotto and the painter of a portrait of Petrarch's Laura, now preserved in the Laurentian library, which earned him two sonnets of eulogy. It is also two Sienese painters who have made the gayest thing in this room, the predella, No. 1304, by Neroccio di Siena (1447-1500) and Francesco di Giorgio di Siena (1439-1502), containing scenes in the life of S. Benedetto. Neroccio did the landscape and figures; the other the architecture, and very fine it is. Another delightful predella is that by Benozzo Gozzoli (1420-1498), Fra Angelico's pupil, whom we have seen at the Riccardi palace. Gozzoli's predella is No. 1302. Finally, look at No. 64, which shows how prettily certain imitators of Fra Angelico could paint.

After the Sala di Lorenzo Monaco let us enter the first Tuscan room. The draughtsmanship of the great Last Judgment fresco by Fra Bartolommeo (1475-1517) and Mariotto Albertinelli (1474-1515) is very fine. It is now a ruin, but enough remains to show that it must have been impressive. These collaborators, although intimate friends, ultimately went different ways, for Fra Bartolommeo came under the influence of Savonarola, burned his nude drawings, and entered the Convent of S. Marco; whereas Albertinelli, who was a convivial follower of Venus, tiring of art and even more of art jargon, took an inn outside the S. Gallo gate and a tavern on the Ponte Vecchio, remarking that he had found a way of life that needed no knowledge of muscles, foreshortening, or perspective, and better still, was without critics. Among his pupils was Franciabigio, whose lovely Madonna of the Well we are coming to in the Tribuna.

Chief among the other pictures are two by the delightful Alessio Baldovinetti, the master of Domenico Ghirlandaio, Nos. 60 and 56; and a large early altar-piece by the brothers Orcagna, painted in 1367 for S. Maria Nuova, now the principal hospital of Florence and once the home of many beautiful pictures. This work is rather dingy now, but it is interesting as coming in part from the hand that designed the tabernacle in Or San Michele and the Loggia de' Lanzi. Another less-known painter represented here is Francesco Granacci (1469-1543), the author of Nos. 1541 and 1280, both rich and warm and pleasing. Granacci was a fellow-pupil of Michelangelo both in Lorenzo de' Medici's garden and in Ghirlandaio's workshop, and the bosom friend of that great man all his life. Like Piero di Cosimo, Granacci was a great hand at pageantry, and Lorenzo de' Medici kept him busy. He was not dependent upon art for his living, but painted for love of it, and Vasari makes him a very agreeable man.

Here too is Gio. Antonio Sogliani (1492-1544), also a rare painter, with a finely coloured and finely drawn "Disputa," No. 63. This painter seems to have had the same devotion to his master, Lorenzo di Credi, that di Credi had for his master, Verrocchio. Vasari calls Sogliani a worthy religious man who minded his own affairs–a good epitaph. His work is rarely met with in Florence, but he has a large fresco at S. Marco. Lorenzo di Credi (1459-1537) himself has two pretty circular paintings here, of which No. 1528 is particularly sweet: "The Virgin and Child with St. John and Angels," all comfortable and happy in a Tuscan meadow; while on an easel is another circular picture, by Pacchiarotto (1477-1535). This has good colour and twilight beauty, but it does not touch one and is not too felicitously composed. Over the door to the Venetian room is a Cosimo Rosselli with a prettily affectionate Madonna and Child.

From this miscellaneous Tuscan room we pass to the two rooms which contain the Venetian pictures, of which I shall say less than might perhaps be expected, not because I do not intensely admire them but because I feel that the chief space in a Florentine book should be given to Florentine or Tuscan things. As a matter of fact, I find myself when in the Uffizi continually drawn to revisit these walls. The chief treasures are the Titians, the Giorgiones, the Mantegnas, the Carpaccio, and the Bellini allegory. These alone would make the Uffizi a Mecca of connoisseurs. Giorgione is to be found in his richest perfection at the Pitti, in his one unforgettable work that is preserved there, but here he is wonderful too, with his Cavalier of Malta, black and golden, and the two rich scenes, Nos. 621 and 630, nominally from Scripture, but really from romantic Italy. To me these three pictures are the jewels of the Venetian collection. To describe them is impossible: enough to say that some glowing genius produced them; and whatever the experts admit, personally I prefer to consider that genius Giorgione. Giorgione, who was born in 1477 and died young–at thirty-three–was, like Titian, the pupil of Bellini, but was greatly influenced by Leonardo da Vinci. Later he became Titian's master. He was passionately devoted to music and to ladies, and it was indeed from a lady that he had his early death, for he continued to kiss her after she had taken the plague. (No bad way to die, either; for to be in the power of an emotion that sways one to such foolishness is surely better than to live the lukewarm calculating lives of most of us.) Giorgione's claim to distinction is that not only was he a glorious colourist and master of light and shade, but may be said to have invented small genre pictures that could be earned about and hung in this or that room at pleasure–such pictures as many of the best Dutch painters were to bend their genius to almost exclusively–his favourite subjects being music parties and picnics. These Moses and Solomon pictures in the Uffizi are of course only a pretext for gloriously coloured arrangements of people with rich scenic backgrounds. No.621 is the finer. The way in which the baby is being held in the other indicates how little Giorgione thought of verisimilitude. The colour was the thing.

After the Giorgiones the Titians, chief of which is No.633, "The Madonna and Child with S. John and S. Anthony," sometimes called the "Madonna of the Roses," a work which throws a pallor over all Tuscan pictures; No.626, the golden Flora, who glows more gloriously every moment (whom we shall see again, at the Pitti, as the Magdalen); the Duke and Duchess of Urbino, Nos.605 and 599, the Duchess set at a window with what looks so curiously like a deep blue Surrey landscape through it and a village spire in the midst; and 618, an unfinished Madonna and Child in which the Master's methods can be followed. The Child, completed save for the final bath of light, is a miracle of draughtsmanship.

The triptych by Andrea Mantegna (1431-1506) is of inexhaustible interest, for here, as ever, Mantegna is full of thought and purpose. The left panel represents the Ascension, Christ being borne upwards by eleven cherubim in a solid cloud; the right panel–by far the best, I think–shows the Circumcision, where the painter has set himself various difficulties of architecture and goldsmith's work for the pleasure of overcoming them, every detail being painted with Dutch minuteness and yet leaving the picture big; while the middle panel, which is concave, depicts an Adoration of the Magi that will bear much study. The whole effect is very northern: not much less so than our own new National Gallery Mabuse. Mantegna also has a charming Madonna and Child, No. 1025, with pleasing pastoral and stone-quarrying activities in the distance.

On the right of the triptych is the so-called Carpaccio (1450-1519), a confused but glorious melee of youths and halberds, reds and yellows and browns, very modern and splendid and totally unlike anything else in the whole gallery. Uccello may possibly be recalled, but only for subject. Finally there is Giovanni Bellini (1426-1516), master of Titian and Giorgione, with his "Sacra Conversazione," No. 631, which means I know not what but has a haunting quality. Later we shall see a picture by Michelangelo which has been accused of blending Christianity and paganism; but Bellini's sole purpose was to do this. We have children from a Bacchic vase and the crowned Virgin; two naked saints and a Venetian lady; and a centaur watching a hermit. The foreground is a mosaic terrace; the background is rocks and water. It is all bizarre and very curious and memorable and quite unique. For the rest, I should mention two charming Guardis; a rich little Canaletto; a nice scene of sheep by Jacopo Bassano; the portrait of an unknown young man by an unknown painter, No. 1157; and Tintoretto's daring "Abraham and Isaac".

The other Venetian room is almost wholly devoted to portraits, chief among them being a red-headed Tintoretto burning furiously, No. 613, and Titian's sly and sinister Caterina Cornaro in her gorgeous dress, No. 648; Piombo's "L'Uomo Ammalato"; Tintoretto's Jacopo Sansovino, the sculptor, the grave old man holding his calipers who made that wonderful Greek Bacchus at the Bargello; Schiavone's ripe, bearded "Ignoto," No. 649, and, perhaps above all, the Moroni, No. 386, black against grey. There is also Paolo Veronese's "Holy Family with S. Catherine," superbly masterly and golden but suggesting the Rialto rather than Nazareth.

One picture gives the next room, the Sala di Michelangelo, its name; but entering from the Venetian room we come first on the right to a very well-known Lippo Lippi, copied in every picture shop in Florence: No. 1307, a Madonna and two Children. Few pictures are so beset by delighted observers, but apart from the perfection of it as an early painting, leaving nothing to later dexterity, its appeal to me is weak. The Madonna (whose head-dress, as so often in Lippo Lippi, foreshadows Botticelli) and the landscape equally delight; the children almost repel, and the decorative furniture in the corner quite repels. The picture is interesting also for its colour, which is unlike anything else in the gallery, the green of the Madonna's dress being especially lovely and distinguished, and vulgarizing the Ghirlandaio–No. 1297–which hangs next. This picture is far too hot throughout, and would indeed be almost displeasing but for the irradiation of the Virgin's face. The other Ghirlandaio–No. 1295–in this room is far finer and sweeter; but at the Accademia and the Badia we are to see him at his best in this class of work. None the less, No. 1295 is a charming thing, and the little Mother and her happy Child, whose big toe is being so reverently adored by the ancient mage, are very near real simple life. This artist, we shall see, always paints healthy, honest babies. The seaport in the distance is charming too.

Ghirlandaio's place in this room is interesting on account of his relation to Michelangelo as first instructor; but by the time that the great master's "Holy Family," hanging here, was painted all traces of Ghirlandaio's influence had disappeared, and if any forerunner is noticeable it is Luca Signorelli. But we must first glance at the pretty little Lorenzo di Credi, No. 1160, the Annunciation, an artificial work full of nice thoughts and touches, with the prettiest little blue Virgin imaginable, a heavenly landscape, and a predella in monochrome, in one scene of which Eve rises from the side of the sleeping Adam with extraordinary realism. The announcing Gabriel is deferential but positive; Mary is questioning but not wholly surprised. In any collection of Annunciations this picture would find a prominent place.

The "Holy Family" of Michelangelo–No. 1139–is remarkable for more than one reason. It is, to begin with, the only finished easel picture that exists from his brush. It is also his one work in oils, for he afterwards despised that medium as being fit "only for children". The frame is contemporary and was made for it, the whole being commissioned by Angelo Doni, a wealthy connoisseur whose portrait by Raphael we shall see in the Pitti, and who, according to Vasari, did his best to get it cheaper than his bargain, and had in the end to pay dearer. The period of the picture is about 1503, while the great David was in progress, when the painter was twenty-eight. That it is masterly and superb there can be no doubt, but, like so much of Michelangelo's work, it suffers from its author's greatness. There is an austerity of power here that ill consorts with the tender domesticity of the scene, and the Child is a young Hercules. The nude figures in the background introduce an alien element and suggest the conflict between Christianity and paganism, the new religion and the old: in short, the Twilight of the Gods. Whether Michelangelo intended this we shall not know; but there it is. The prevailing impression left by the picture is immense power and virtuosity and no religion. In the beautiful Luca Signorelli–No.74–next it, we find at once a curious similarity and difference. The Madonna and Child only are in the foreground, a not too radiant but very tender couple; in the background are male figures nearly nude: not quite, as Michelangelo made them, and suggesting no discord as in his picture. Luca was born in 1441, and was thus thirty-four years older than Michelangelo. This picture is perhaps that one presented by Luca to Lorenzo de' Medici, of which Vasari tells, and if so it was probably on a wall in the Medici palace when Michelangelo as a boy was taught with Lorenzo's sons. Luca's sweetness was alien to Michelangelo, but not his melancholy or his sense of composition; while Luca's devotion to the human form as the unit of expression was in Michelangelo carried out to its highest power. Vasari, who was a relative of Luca's and a pupil of Michelangelo's, says that his master had the greatest admiration for Luca's genius.

Luca Signorelli was born at Cortona, and was instructed by Piero della Francesca, whose one Uffizi painting is in a later room. His chief work is at Cortona, at Rome (in the Sixtine Chapel), and at Orvieto. His fame was sufficient in

Florence in 1491 for him to be made one of the judges of the designs for the façade of the Duomo. Luca lived to a great age, not dying till 1524, and was much beloved. He was magnificent in his habits and loved fine clothes, was very kindly and helpful in disposition, and the influence of his naturalness and sincerity upon art was great. One very pretty sad story is told of him, to the effect that when his son, whom he had dearly loved, was killed at Cortona, he caused the body to be stripped, and painted it with the utmost exactitude, that through his own handiwork he might be able to contemplate that treasure of which fate had robbed him. Perhaps the most beautiful or at any rate the most idiosyncratic thing in the picture before us is its lovely profusion of wayside flowers. These come out but poorly in the photograph, but in the painting they are exquisite both in form and in detail. Luca painted them as if he loved them. (There is a hint of the same thoughtful care in the flowers in No. 1133, by Luca, in our National Gallery; but these at Florence are the best.) No. 74 is in tempera: the next, also by Luca, No.1291, is in oil, a "Holy Family," a work at once powerful, rich, and sweet. Here, again, we may trace an influence on Michelangelo, for the child is shown deprecating a book which his mother is displaying, while in the beautiful marble tondo of the "Madonna and Child" by Michelangelo, which we are soon to see in the Bargello, a reading lesson is in progress, and the child wearying of it. We find Luca again in the next large picture–No.1547–a Crucifixion, with various Saints, done in collaboration with Perugino. The design suggests Luca rather than his companion, and the woman at the foot of the cross is surely the type of which he was so fond. The drawing of Christ is masterly and all too sombre for Perugino. Finally, there is a Luca predella, No. 1298, representing the Annunciation, the Birth of Christ (in which Joseph is older almost than in any version), and the Adoration of the Magi, all notable for freedom and richness. Note the realism and charm and the costume of the two pages of the Magi.

And now we come to what is perhaps the most lovely picture in the whole gallery, judged purely as colour and sweetness and design–No.1549–a "Madonna

Adoring," with Filippino Lippi's name and an interrogation mark beneath it. Who painted it if not Filippino? That is the question; but into such problems, which confront one at every turn in Florence, I am neither qualified nor anxious to enter. When doctors disagree any one may decide before me. The thought, moreover, that always occurs in the presence of these good debatable pictures, is that any doubt as to their origin merely enriches this already over-rich period, since some one had to paint them. Simon not pure becomes hardly less remarkable than Simon pure.

If only the Baby were more pleasing, this would be perhaps the most delightful picture in the world: as it is, its blues alone lift it to the heavens of delectableness. By an unusual stroke of fortune a crack in the paint where the panels join has made a star in the tender blue sky. The Tuscan landscape is very still and beautiful; the flowers, although conventional and not accurate like Luca's, are as pretty as can be; the one unsatisfying element is the Baby, who is a little clumsy and a little in pain, but diffuses radiance none the less. And the Mother–the Mother is all perfection and winsomeness. Her face and hands are exquisite, and the Tuscan twilight behind her is so lovely. I have given a reproduction, but colour is essential.

The remaining three pictures in the room are a Bastiano and a Pollaiolo, which are rather for the student than for the wanderer, and a charming Ignoto, No. 75, which I like immensely. But Ignoto nearly always paints well.

In the Sala di Leonardo are two pictures which bear the name of this most fascinating of all the painters of the world. One is the Annunciation, No. 1288, upon the authenticity of which much has been said and written, and the other an unfinished Adoration of the Magi which cannot be questioned by anyone. The probabilities are that the Annunciation is an early work and that the ascription is accurate: at Oxford is a drawing known to be Leonardo's that is almost certainly a study for a detail of this work, while among the Leonardo drawings in the His de la Salle collection at the Louvre is something very like a first sketch of the whole. Certainly one can think of no one else who could have given the picture its quality, which increases in richness with every visit to the gallery; but the workshop of Verrocchio, where Leonardo worked, together with Lorenzo di Credi and Perugino, with Andrea of the True Eye over all, no doubt put forth wonderful things. The Annunciation is unique in the collection, both in colour and character: nothing in the Uffizi so deepens. There are no cypresses like these in any other picture, no finer drawing than that of Mary's hands. Luca's flowers are better, in the adjoining room; one is not too happy about the pedestal of the reading-desk; and there are Virgins whom we can like more; but as a whole it is perhaps the most fascinating picture of all, for it has the Leonardo darkness as well as light.

Of Leonardo I could write for ever, but this book is not the place; for though he was a Florentine, Florence has very little of his work: these pictures only, and one of these only for certain, together with an angel in a work by Verrocchio at the Accademia which we shall see, and possibly a sculptured figure over the north door of the Baptistery. Ludovico Sforza, Duke of Milan, and Francis I of France, lured him away, to the eternal loss of his own city. It is Milan and Paris that are richest in his work, and after that London, which has at South Kensington a sculptured relief by him as well as a painting at the National Gallery, a cartoon at Burlington House, and the British Museum drawings.

His other work here–No. 1252–in the grave brown frame, was to have been Leonardo's greatest picture in oil, so Vasari says: larger, in fact, than any known picture at that time. Being very indistinct, it is, curiously enough, best as the light begins to fail and the beautiful wistful faces emerge from the gloom. In their presence one recalls Leonardo's remark in one of his notebooks that faces are most interesting beneath a troubled sky. "You should make your portrait," he adds, "at the hour of the fall of the evening when it is cloudy or misty, for the light then is perfect." In the background one can discern the prancing horses of the Magi's suite; a staircase with figures ascending and descending; the rocks and trees of Tuscany; and looking at it one cannot but ponder upon the fatality which seems to have pursued this divine and magical genius, ordaining that almost everything that he put forth should be either destroyed or unfinished: his work in the Castello at Milan, which might otherwise be an eighth wonder of the world, perished; his "Last Supper" at Milan perishing; his colossal equestrian statue of Francesco Sforza broken to pieces; his sculpture lost; his Palazzo Vecchio battle cartoon perished; this picture only a sketch. Even after long years the evil fate still persists, for in 1911 his "Gioconda" was stolen from the Louvre by madman or knave.

Among the other pictures in this room is the rather hot "Adoration of the Magi," by Cosimo Rosselli (1439-1507), over the Leonardo "Annunciation," a glowing scene of colour and animation: this Cosimo being the Cosimo from whom Piero di Cosimo took his name, and an associate of Botticelli, Ghirlandaio, Perugino, and Luca Signorelli on the Sixtine Chapel frescoes. On the left wall is Uccello's battle piece, No. 52, very like that in our National Gallery: rich and glorious as decoration, but quite bearing out Vasari's statement that Uccello could not draw horses. Uccello was a most laborious student of animal life and so absorbed in the mysteries of perspective that he preferred them to bed; but he does not seem to have been able to unite them. He was a perpetual butt of Donatello. It is told of him that having a commission to paint a fresco for the Mercato Vecchio he kept the progress of the work a secret and allowed no one to see it. At last, when it was finished, he drew aside the sheet for Donatello, who was buying fruit, to admire. "Ah, Paolo," said the sculptor reproachfully, "now that you ought to be covering it up, you uncover it."

There remain a superb nude study of Venus by Lorenzo di Credi, No. 3452–one of the pictures which escaped Savonarola's bonfire of vanities, and No. 1305, a Virgin and Child with various Saints by Domenico Veneziano (1400-1461), who taught Gentile da Fabriano, the teacher of Jacopo Bellini. This picture is a complete contrast to the Uccello: for that is all tapestry, richness, and belligerence, and this is so pale and gentle, with its lovely light green, a rare colour in this gallery.

CHAPTER X

THE Uffizi III: Botticelli

A painter apart–Sandro Filipepi–Artists' names–Piero de' Medici–The "Adoration of the Magi"–The "Judith" pictures–Lucrezia Tornabuoni, Lorenzo and Giuliano's mother–The Tournaments–The "Birth of Venus" and the "Primavera"–Simonetta–A new star–Sacred pictures–Savonarola and "The Calumny"–The National Gallery–Botticelli's old age and death.

We come next to the Sala di Botticelli, and such is the position held by this painter in the affection of visitors to Florence, and such the wealth of works from his hand that the Uffizi possesses, that I feel that a single chapter may well be devoted to his genius, more particularly as many of his pictures were so closely associated with Piero de' Medici and Lorenzo de' Medici. We see Botticelli here at his most varied. The Accademia also is very rich in his work, having above all the "Primavera," and in this chapter I shall glance at the Accademia pictures too, returning to them when we reach that gallery in due course. Among the great Florentine masters Botticelli stands apart by reason not only of the sensitive wistful delicacy of his work, but for the profound interest of his personality. He is not essentially more beautiful than his friend Filippino Lippi or–occasionally–than Fra Lippo Lippi his master;

but he is always deeper. One feels that he too felt the emotion that his characters display; he did not merely paint, he thought and suffered. Hence his work is dramatic. Again Botticelli had far wider sympathies than most of his contemporaries. He was a friend of the Medici, a neo-Platonist, a student of theology with the poet Palmieri, an illustrator of Dante, and a devoted follower of Savonarola. Of the part that women played in his life we know nothing: in fact we know less of him intimately than of almost any of the great painters; but this we may guess, that he was never a happy man. His work falls naturally into divisions corresponding to his early devotion to Piero de' Medici and his wife Lucrezia Tornabuoni, in whose house for a while he lived; to his interest in their sons Lorenzo and Giuliano; and finally to his belief in Savonarola. Sublime he never is; comforting he never is; but he is everything else. One can never forget in his presence the tragedy that attends the too earnest seeker after beauty: not "all is vanity" does Botticelli say, but "all is transitory".

Botticelli, as we now call him, was the son of Mariano Filipepi and was born in Florence in 1447. According to one account he was called Sandro di Botticelli because he was apprenticed to a goldsmith of that name; according to another his brother Antonio, a goldsmith, was known as Botticello (which means a little barrel), and Sandro being with him was called Sandro di Botticello. Whatever the cause, the fact remains that the name of Filipepi is rarely used.

And here a word as to the capriciousness of the nomenclature of artists. We know some by their Christian names; some by their surnames; some by their nicknames; some by the names of their towns, and some by the names of their masters. Tommaso Bigordi, a goldsmith, was so clever in designing a pretty garland for women's hair that he was called Ghirlandaio, the garland-maker, and his painter son Domenico is therefore known for ever as Uomenico Ghirlandaio. Paolo Doni, a painter of battle scenes, was so fond of birds that he was known as Uccello (a bird) and now has no other name; Pietro Vannucci coming from Perugia was called Perugino; Agnolo di

Francesco di Migliore happened to be a tailor with a genius of a son, Andrea; that genius is therefore Andrea of the Tailor–del Sarto–for all time. And so forth.

To return to Botticelli. In 1447, when he was born, Fra Angelico was sixty; and Masaccio had been dead for some years. At the age of twelve the boy was placed with Fra Lippo Lippi, then a man of a little more than fifty, to learn painting. That Lippo was his master one may see continually, but particularly by comparison of his headdresses with almost any of Botticelli's. Both were minutely careful in this detail. But where Lippo was beautifully obvious, Sandro was beautifully analytical: he was also, as I have said, much more interesting and dramatic.

Botticelli's best patron was Piero de' Medici, who took him into his house, much as his son Lorenzo was to take Michelangelo into his, and made him one of the family. For Piero, Botticelli always had affection and respect, and when he painted his "Fortitude" as one of the Pollaiuoli's series of the Virtues for the Mercatanzia (of which several are in this gallery), he made the figure symbolize Piero's life and character–or so it is possible, if one wishes to believe. But it should be understood that almost nothing is known about Botticelli and the origin of his pictures. At Piero's request Botticelli painted the "Adoration of the Magi" (No. 1286) which was to hang in S. Maria Novella as an offering of gratitude for Piero's escape from the conspiracy of Luca Pitti in 1466. Piero had but just succeeded to Cosimo when Pitti, considering him merely an invalid, struck his blow. By virtue largely of the young Lorenzo's address the attack miscarried: hence the presence of Lorenzo in the picture, on the extreme left, with a sword. Piero himself in scarlet kneels in the middle; Giuliano, his second son, doomed to an early death by assassination, is kneeling on his right. The picture is not only a sacred painting but (like the Gozzoli fresco at the Riccardi palace) an exaltation of the Medici family. The dead Cosimo is at the Child's feet; the dead Giovanni, Piero's brother, stands close to the kneeling Giuliano. Among the other persons represented are collateral Medici and certain of their friends.

It is by some accepted that the figure in yellow, on the extreme right, looking out of this picture, is Botticelli himself. But for a portrait of the painter of more authenticity we must go to the Carmine, where, in the Brancacci chapel, we shall see a fresco by Botticelli's friend Filippino Lippi representing the Crucifixion of S. Peter, in which our painter is depicted on the right, looking on at the scene–a rather coarse heavy face, with a large mouth and long hair. He wears a purple cap and red cloak. Vasari tells us that Botticelli, although so profoundly thoughtful and melancholy in his work, was extravagant, pleasure loving, and given to practical jokes. Part at least of this might be gathered from observation of Filippino Lippi's portrait of him. According to Vasari it was No. 1286 which brought Botticelli his invitation to Rome from Sixtus IV to decorate the Sixtine Chapel. But that was several years later and much was to happen in the interval.

The two little "Judith" pictures (Nos. 1156 and 1158) were painted for Piero de' Medici and had their place in the Medici palace. In 1494, when Piero di Lorenzo de' Medici was banished from Florence and the palace looted, they were stolen and lost sight of; but during the reign of Francis I they reappeared and were presented to his wife Bianca Capella and once more placed with the Medici treasures. No. 1156, the Judith walking springily along, sword in hand, having slain the tyrant, is one of the masterpieces of paint. Everything about it is radiant, superb, and unforgettable.

One other picture which the young painter made for his patron–or in this case his patroness, Lucrezia Tornabuoni, Piero's wife–is the "Madonna of the Magnificat," No. 1267, with its beautiful children and sweet Madonna, its lovely landscape but not too attractive Child. The two boys are Lorenzo, on the left, and Giuliano, in yellow. One of their sisters leans over them. Here the boys are perhaps, in Botticelli's way, typified rather than portrayed. Although this picture came so early in his career Botticelli never excelled its richness, beauty, and depth of feeling, nor its liquid delicacy of treatment. Lucrezia Tornabuoni, for whom he painted it, was a very remarkable woman, not only a good mother to her children and a good wife to Piero, but a poet and exemplar. She survived Piero by thirteen years and her son Giuliano by five. Botticelli painted her portrait, which is now in Berlin.

These pictures are the principal work of Botticelli's first period, which coincides with the five years of Piero's rule and the period of mourning for him.

He next appears in what many of his admirers find his most fascinating mood, as a joyous allegorist, the picture of Venus rising from the sea in this room, the "Primavera" which we shall see at the Accademia, and the "Mars and Venus" in our National Gallery, belonging to this epoch. But in order to understand them we must again go to history. Piero was succeeded in 1469 by his son Lorenzo the Magnificent, who continued his father's friendship for the young painter, now twenty-two years of age. In 1474 Lorenzo devised for his brother Giuliano a tournament in the Piazza of S. Croce very like that which Piero had given for Lorenzo on the occasion of his betrothal in 1469; and Botticelli was commissioned by Lorenzo to make pictures commemorating the event. Verrocchio again helped with the costumes; Lucrezia Donati again was Queen of the Tournament; but the Queen of Beauty was the sixteen-year-old bride of Marco Vespucci–the lovely Simonetta Cattaneo, a lady greatly beloved by all and a close friend both of Giuliano and Lorenzo.

The praises of Lorenzo's tournament had been sung by Luca Pulci: Giuliano's were sung by Poliziano, under the title "La Giostra di Giuliano de' Medici," and it is this poem which Botticelli may be said to have illustrated, for both poet and artist employ the same imagery. Thus Poliziano, or Politian (of whom we shall hear more in the chapter on S. Marco) compares Simonetta to Venus, and in stanzas 100 and 101 speaks of her birth, describing her blown to earth over the sea by the breath of the Zephyrs, and welcomed there by the Hours, one of whom offers her a robe. This, Botticelli translates into exquisite tempera with a wealth of pretty thoughts. The cornflowers and daisies on the Hour's dress are alone a perennial joy.

Simonetta as Venus has some of the wistfulness of the Madonnas; and not without reason does Botticelli give her this expression, for her days were very short. In the "Primavera," which we are to see at the Accademia, but which must be described here, we find Simonetta again but we do not see her first. We see first that slender upright commanding figure, all flowers and youth and conquest, in her lovely floral dress, advancing over the grass like thistle-down. Never before in painting had anything been done at once so distinguished and joyous and pagan as this. For a kindred emotion one had to go to Greek sculpture, but Botticelli, while his grace and joy are Hellenic, was intensely modern too: the problems of the Renaissance, the tragedy of Christianity, equally cloud his brow.

The symbolism of the "Primavera" is interesting. Glorious Spring is returning to earth–in the presence of Venus–once more to make all glad, and with her her attendants to dance and sing, and the Zephyrs to bring the soft breezes; and by Spring Botticelli meant the reign of Lorenzo, whose tournament motto was "Le temps revient". Simonetta is again the central figure, and never did Botticelli paint more exquisitely than here. Her bosom is the prettiest in Florence; the lining of her robe over her right arm has such green and blue and gold as never were seen elsewhere; her golden sandals are delicate as gossamer. Over her head a little cupid hovers, directing his arrow at Mercury, on the extreme left, beside the three Graces.

In Mercury, who is touching the trees with his caduceus and bidding them burgeon, some see Giuliano de' Medici, who was not yet betrothed. But when the picture was painted both Giuliano and Simonetta were dead: Simonetta first, of consumption, in 1476, and Giuliano, by stabbing in 1478. Lorenzo, who was at Pisa during Simonetta's illness, detailed his own physician for her care. On hearing of her death he walked out into the night and noticed for the first time a brilliant star. "See," he said, "either the soul of that most gentle lady hath been transferred into that new star or else hath it been joined together thereunto." Of Giuliano's end we have read in Chapter II, and it was Botticelli, whose destinies were so closely bound up with the Medici, who was commissioned to paint portraits of the murderous Pazzi to be displayed outside the Palazzo Vecchio.

A third picture in what may be called the tournament period is found by some in the "Venus and Mars," No. 915, in our National Gallery. Here Giuliano would be Mars, and Venus either one woman in particular whom Florence wished him to marry, or all women, typified by one, trying to lure him from other pre-occupations, such as hunting. To make her Simonetta is to go too far; for she is not like the Simonetta of the other pictures, and Simonetta was but recently married and a very model of fair repute. In No. 916 in the National Gallery is a "Venus with Cupids" (which might be by Botticelli and might be by that interesting painter of whom Mr. Berenson has written so attractively as Amico di Sandro), in which Politian's description of Venus, in his poem, is again closely followed.

After the tournament pictures we come in Botticelli's career to the Sixtine Chapel frescoes, and on his return to Florence to other frescoes, including that lovely one at the Villa Lemmi (then the Villa Tornabuoni) which is now on the staircase of the Louvre. These are followed by at least two more Medici pictures–the portrait of Piero di Lorenzo de' Medici, in this room, No. 1154, the sad-faced youth with the medal; and the "Pallas and the Centaur" at the Pitti, an historical record of Lorenzo's success as a diplomatist when he went to Naples in 1480.

The latter part of Botticelli's life was spent under the influence of Savonarola and in despair at the wickedness of the world and its treatment of that prophet. His pictures became wholly religious, but it was religion without joy. Never capable of disguising the sorrow that underlies all human happiness–or, as I think of it in looking at his work, the sense of transience–Botticelli, as age came upon him, was more than ever depressed. One has the feeling that he was persuaded that only through devotion and self-negation could peace of mind be gained, and yet for himself could find none. The sceptic was too strong in him. Savonarola's eloquence could not make him serene, however much he may have come beneath its spell. It but served to increase his melancholy. Hence these wistful despondent Madonnas, all so conscious of the tragedy before their Child; hence these troubled angels and shadowed saints.

Savonarola was hanged and burned in 1498, and Botticelli paid a last tribute to his friend in the picture in this room called "The Calumny". Under the pretence of merely illustrating a passage in Lucian, who was one of his favourite authors, Botticelli has represented the campaign against the great reformer. The hall represents Florence; the judge (with the ears of an ass) the Signoria and the Pope. Into these ears Ignorance and Suspicion are whispering. Calumny, with Envy at her side and tended by Fraud and Deception, holds a torch in one hand and with the other drags her victim, who personifies (but with no attempt at a likeness) Savonarola. Behind are the figures of Remorse, cloaked and miserable, and Truth, naked and unafraid. The statues in the niches ironically represent abstract virtues. Everything in the decoration of the palace points to enlightenment and content; and beyond is the calmest and greenest of seas.

One more picture was Botticelli to paint, and this also was to the glory of Savonarola. By good fortune it belongs to the English people and is No. 1034 in the National Gallery. It has upon it a Greek inscription in the painter's own hand which runs in English as follows: "This picture I, Alessandro, painted at the end of the year 1500, in the troubles of Italy, in the half-time after the time during the fulfilment of the eleventh of St. John, in the second woe of the Apocalypse, in the loosing of the devil for three years and a half. Afterwards he shall be confined, and we shall see him trodden down, as in this picture." The loosing of the devil was the three years and a half after Savonarola's execution on May 23rd, 1498, when Florence was mad with reaction from the severity of his discipline. S. John says, "I will give power unto my two witnesses, and they shall prophesy"; the painter makes three, Savonarola having had two comrades with him. The picture was intended to give heart to the followers of Savonarola and bring promise of ultimate triumph.

After the death of Savonarola, Botticelli became both poor and infirm. He had saved no money and all his friends were dead–Piero de' Medici, Lorenzo, Giuliano, Lucrezia, Simonetta, Filippino Lippi, and Savonarola. He hobbled about on crutches for a while, a pensioner of the Medici family, and dying at the age of seventy-eight was buried in Ognissanti, but without a tombstone for fear of desecration by the enemies of Savonarola's adherents.

Such is the outline of Botticelli's life. We will now look at such of the pictures in this room as have not been mentioned.

Entering from the Sala di Leonardo, the first picture on the right is the "Birth of Venus". Then the very typical circular picture–a shape which has come to be intimately associated with this painter–No. 1289, "The Madonna of the Pomegranate," one of his most beautiful works, and possibly yet another designed for Lucrezia Tornabuoni, for the curl on the forehead of the boy to the left of the Madonna–who is more than usually troubled–is very like that for which Giuliano de' Medici was famous. This is a very lovely work, although its colour is a little depressed. Next is the most remarkable of the Piero de' Medici pictures, which I have already touched upon–No. 1286, "The Adoration of the Magi," as different from the Venus as could be: the Venus so cool and transparent, and this so hot and rich, with its haughty Florentines and sumptuous cloaks. Above it is No. 23, a less subtle group–the Madonna, the Child and angels–difficult to see. And then comes the beautiful "Magnificat," which we know to have been painted for Lucrezia Tornabuoni and which shall here introduce a passage from Pater: "For with Botticelli she too, although she holds in her hands the 'Desire of all nations,' is one of those who are neither for Jehovah nor for His enemies; and her choice is on her face. The white light on it is cast up hard and cheerless from below, as when snow lies upon the ground, and the children look up with surprise at the strange whiteness of the ceiling. Her trouble is in the very caress of the mysterious child, whose gaze is always far from her, and who has already that sweet look of devotion which men have never been able altogether to love, and which still makes the born saint an object almost of suspicion to his earthly brethren. Once, indeed, he guides her hand to transcribe in a book the words of her exaltation, the 'Ave,' and the 'Magnificat,' and the 'Gaude Maria,' and the young angels, glad to rouse her for a moment from her devotion, are eager to hold the ink-horn and to support the book. But the pen almost drops from her hand, and the high cold words have no meaning for her, and her true children are those others among whom, in her rude home, the intolerable honour came to her, with that look of wistful inquiry on their irregular faces which you see in startled animals–gipsy children, such as those who, in Apennine villages, still hold out their long brown arms to beg of you, with their thick black hair nicely combed, and fair white linen on their sunburnt throats."

The picture's frame is that which was made for it four hundred and fifty years ago: by whom, I cannot say, but it was the custom at that time for the painter himself to be responsible also for the frame.

The glory of the end wall is the "Annunciation," reproduced in this book. The picture is a work that may perhaps not wholly please at first, the cause largely of the vermilion on the floor, but in the end conquers. The hands are among the most beautiful in existence, and the landscape, with its one tree and its fairy architecture, is a continual delight. Among "Annunciations," as among pictures, it stands very high. It has more of sophistication than most: the Virgin not only recognizes the honour, but the doom, which the painter himself foreshadows in the predella, where Christ is seen rising from the grave. None of Fra Angelico's simple radiance here, and none of Fra Lippo Lippi's glorified matter-of-fact. Here is tragedy. The painting of the Virgin's head-dress is again marvellous.

Next the "Annunciation" on the left is, to my eyes, one of Botticelli's most attractive works: No. 1303, just the Madonna and Child again, in a niche, with roses climbing behind them: the Madonna one of his youngest, and more placid and simple than most, with more than a hint of the Verrocchio type in her face. To the "School of Botticelli" this is sometimes attributed: it may be rightly. Its pendant is another "Madonna and Child," No. 76, more like Lippo Lippi and very beautiful in its darker graver way.

The other wall has the "Fortitude," the "Calumny," and the two little "Judith and Holofernes" pictures. Upon the "Fortitude," to which I have already alluded, it is well to look at Ruskin, who, however, was not aware that the artist intended any symbolic reference to the character and career of Piero de' Medici. The criticism is in "Mornings in Florence" and it is followed by some fine pages on the "Judith". The "Justice," "Prudence," and "Charity" of the Pollaiuolo brothers, belonging to the same series as the "Fortitude," are also here; but after the "Fortitude" one does not look at them.

CHAPTER XI

HE Uffizi IV: Remaining Rooms

t
S. Zenobius–Piero della Francesca–Federigo da Montefeltro–Melozzo da Forli–The Tribuna–Raphael–Re-arrangement–The gems–The self-painted portraits–A northern room–Hugo van der Goes– Tommaso Portinari–The sympathetic Memling–Rubens riotous–Vittoria della Rovere–Baroccio–Honthors Giovanni the indiscreet–The Medusa–Medici miniatures–Hercules Seghers–The Sala di Niobe– Beautiful antiques.

Passing from the Sala di Botticelli through the Sala di Lorenzo Monaco and the first Tuscan rooms to the corridor, we come to the second Tuscan room, which is dominated by Andrea del Sarto (1486-1531), whose "Madonna and Child," with "S. Francis and S. John the Evangelist"–No. 112–is certainly the favourite picture here, as it is, in reproduction, in so many homes; but, apart from the Child, I like far better the "S. Giacomo"–No. 1254–so sympathetic and rich in colour, which is reproduced in this volume. Another good Andrea is No. 93–a soft and misty apparition of Christ to the Magdalen. The Sodoma (1477-1549) on the easel–"S. Sebastian," No. 1279–is very beautiful in its Leonardesque hues and romantic landscape, and the two Ridolfo Ghirlandaios (1483-1561) near it are interesting as representing, with much hard force, scenes in the story of S. Zenobius, of Florence, of whom we read in chapter II. In one he restores life to the dead child in the midst of a Florentine crowd; in the other his bier, passing the Baptistery, reanimates the dead tree. Giotto's tower and the tower of the Palazzo Vecchio are to be seen on the left. A very different picture is the Cosimo Rosselli, No. 1280 his, a comely "Madonna and Saints," with a motherly thought in the treatment of the bodice.

Among the other pictures is a naked sprawling scene of bodies and limbs by Cosimo I's favourite painter, Bronzino (1502-1572), called "The Saviour in Hell," and two nice Medici children from the same brush, which was kept busy both on the living and ancestral lineaments of that family; two Filippino Lippis, both fine if with a little too much colour for this painter: one–No. 1257–approaching the hotness of a Ghirlandaio carpet piece, but a great feat of crowded activity; the other, No. 1268, having a beautiful blue Madonna and a pretty little cherub with a red book. Piero di Cosimo is here, religious and not mythological; and here are a very straightforward and satisfying Mariotto Albertinelli–the "Virgin and S. Elizabeth," very like a Fra Bartolommeo; a very rich and beautiful "Deposition" by Botticini, one of Verrocchio's pupils, with a gay little predella underneath it, and a pretty "Holy Family" by Franciabigio. But Andrea remains the king of the walls.

From this Sala a little room is gained which I advise all tired visitors to the Uffizi to make their harbour of refuge and recuperation; for it has only three or four pictures in it and three or four pieces of sculpture and some pleasant maps and tapestry on the walls, and from its windows you look across the brown-red tiles to S. Miniato. The pictures, although so few, are peculiarly attractive, being the work of two very rare hands, Piero della Francesca (? 1398-1492) and Melozzo da Forli (1438-1494). Melozzo has here a very charming Annunciation in two panels, the fascination of which I cannot describe. That they are fascinating there is, however, no doubt. We have symbolical figures by him in our National Gallery–again hanging next to Piero della Francesca–but they are not the equal of these in charm, although very charming. These grow more attractive with every visit: the eager advancing angel with his lily, and the timid little Virgin in her green dress, with folded hands.

The two Pieros are, of course, superb. Piero never painted anything that was not distinguished and liquid, and here he gives us of his best: portraits of Federigo da Montefeltro, Duke of Urbino, and Battista, his second Duchess, with classical scenes behind them. Piero della Francesca has ever been one of my favourite painters, and here he is wholly a joy. Of his works Florence has but few, since he was not a Florentine, nor did he work here, being engaged chiefly at Urbino, Ferrara, Arezzo, and Rome. His life ended sadly, for he became totally blind. In addition to his painting he was a mathematician of much repute. The Duke of Urbino here depicted is Federigo da Montefeltro, who ruled from 1444 to 1482, and in 1459 married as his second wife a daughter of Alessandro Sforza, of Pesaro, the wedding being the occasion of Piero's pictures. The duke stands out among the many Italian lords of that time as a humane and beneficent ruler and collector, and eager to administer well. He was a born fighter, and it was owing to the loss of his right eye and the fracture of his noble old nose that he is seen here in such a determined profile against the lovely light over the Umbrian hills. The symbolical chariots in the landscape at the back represent respectively the Triumph of Fame (the Duke's) and the Triumph of Chastity (that of the Duchess). The Duke's companions are Victory, Prudence, Fortitude, Justice, and Temperance; the little Duchess's are Love, Hope, Faith, Charity, and Innocence; and if these are not exquisite pictures I never saw any.

The statues in the room should not be missed, particularly the little Genius of Love, the Bacchus and Ampelos, and the spoilt little comely boy supposed to represent–and quite conceivably–the infant Nero.

Crossing the large Tuscan room again, we come to a little narrow room filled with what are now called cabinet pictures: far too many to study properly, but comprising a benignant old man's head, No. 1167, which is sometimes called a Filippino Lippi and sometimes a Masaccio, a fragment of a fresco;

a boy from the serene perfect hand of Perugino, No. 1217; two little panels by Fra Bartolommeo–No. 1161–painted for a tabernacle to hold a Donatello relief and representing the Circumcision and Nativity, in colours, and at the back a pretty Annunciation in monochrome; No. 1235, on the opposite wall, a very sweet Mother and Child by the same artist; a Perseus liberating Andromeda, by Piero di Cosimo, No. 1312; two or three Lorenzo di Credis; two or three Alloris; a portrait of Galeazzo Maria Sforza, by Antonio Pollaiuolo; and three charming little scenes from the lives of S. John the Baptist and the Virgin, by Fra Angelico, which belong properly to the predella of an altarpiece that we saw in the first room we entered–No. 1290, "The Coronation of the Virgin". No. 1162 has the gayest green dress in it imaginable.

And here we enter the Tribuna, which is to the Uffizi what the Salon Carré is to the Louvre: the special treasure-room of the gallery, holding its most valuable pictures. But to-day there are as good works outside it as in; for the Michelangelo has been moved to another room, and Botticelli (to name no other) is not represented here at all. Probably the statue famous as the Venus de' Medici would be considered the Tribuna's chief possession; but not by me. Nor should I vote either for Titian's Venus. In sculpture I should choose rather the "Knife-sharpener," and among the pictures Raphael's "Madonna del Cardellino," No. 1129. But this is not to suggest that everything is not a masterpiece, for it is. Beginning at the door leading from the room of the little pictures, we find, on our left, Raphael's "Ignota," No. 1120, so rich and unfeeling, and then Francia's portrait of Evangelista Scappi, so rich and real and a picture that one never forgets. Raphael's Julius II comes next, not so powerful as the version in the Pitti, and above that Titian's famous Venus. In Perugino's portrait of Francesco delle Opere, No. 287, we find an evening sky and landscape still more lovely than Francia's. This Francesco was brother of Giovanni delle Corniole, a protégé of Lorenzo de' Medici, famous as a carver of intaglios, whose portrait of Savonarola in this medium, now preserved in the Uffizi, in the Gem Room, was said by Michelangelo to carry art to its farthest possible point.

A placid and typical Perugino–the Virgin and two saints–comes next, and then a northern air sweeps in with Van Dyck's Giovanni di Montfort, now darkening into gloom but very fine and commanding. Titian's second Venus is above, for which his daughter Lavinia acted as model (the Venus of the other version being possibly the Marchesa della Rovere), and under it is the only Luini in the Uffizi, unmistakably from the sweet hand and full of Leonardesque influence. Beneath this is a rich and decorative work of the Veronese school, a portrait of Elisabetta Gonzaga, with another evening sky. Then we go north again, to Dürer's Adoration of the Magi, a picture full of pleasant detail–a little mountain town here, a knight in difficulties with his horse there, two butterflies close to the Madonna–and interesting also for the treatment of the main theme in Dürer's masterly careful way; and then to Spain to Spagnoletto's "S. Jerome" in sombre chiaroscuro; then north again to a painfully real Christ crowned with thorns, by Lucas van Leyden, and the mousy, Reynoldsy, first wife of Peter Paul Rubens, while a Van Dyck portrait under a superb Domenichino and an "Adam and Eve" by Lucas Cranach complete the northern group. And so we come to the two Correggios–so accomplished and rich and untouching–all delightful virtuosity without feeling. The favourite is, of course, No. 1134, for its adorable Baby, whose natural charm atones for its theatrical Mother.

On the other side of the door is No. 1129, the perfect "Madonna del Cardellino" of Raphael, so called from the goldfinch that the little boys are caressing. This, one is forced to consider one of the perfect pictures of the world, even though others may communicate more pleasure. The landscape is so exquisite and the mild sweetness of the whole work so complete; and yet, although the technical mastery is almost thrilling, the "Madonna del Pozzo" by Andrea del Sarto's friend Franciabigio, close by–No. 1125–arouses infinitely livelier feelings in the observer, so much movement and happiness has it. Raphael is perfect but cold; Franciabigio is less perfect (although exceedingly accomplished) but warm with life. The charm of this picture is as notable as the skill of Raphael's: it is wholly joyous, and the little Madonna really once lived. Both are reproduced in this volume.

Raphael's neighbouring youthful "John the Baptist" is almost a Giorgione for richness, but is as truly Raphael as the Sebastian del Piombo, once (like the Franciabigio also) called a Raphael, is not. How it came to be considered Raphael, except that there may be a faint likeness to the Fornarina, is a mystery.

The rooms next the Tribuna have for some time been under reconstruction, and of these I say little, nor of what pictures are to be placed there. But with the Tribuna, in any case, the collection suddenly declines, begins to crumble. The first of these rooms, in the spring of this year, 1912, was opened with a number of small Italian paintings; but they are probably only temporarily there. Chief among them was a Parmigianino, a Boltraffio, a pretty little Guido Reni, a Cosimo Tura, a Lorenzo Costa, but nothing really important.

In the tiny Gem Room at the end of the corridor are wonders of the lapidary's art–and here is the famous intaglio portrait of Savonarola–but they want better treatment. The vases and other ornaments should have the light all round them, as in the Galerie d'Apollon at the Louvre. These are packed together in wall cases and are hard to see.

Passing through the end corridor, where the beautiful Matrona reclines so placidly on her couch against the light, and where we have such pleasant views of the Ponte Vecchio, the Trinita bridge, the Arno, and the Apennines, so fresh and real and soothing after so much paint, we come to the rooms containing the famous collection of self-painted portraits, which, moved hither from Rome, has been accumulating in the Uffizi for many years and is still growing, to be invited to contribute to it being one of the highest honours a painter can receive. The portraits occupy eight rooms and a passage. Though the collection is historically and biographically valuable, it contains for every interesting portrait three or four dull ones, and thus becomes something of a weariness. Among the best are Lucas Cranach, Anton More, Van Dyck, Rembrandt (three), Rubens, Seybold, Jordaens, Reynolds, and Romney, all of which remind us of Michelangelo's dry comment, "Every painter draws himself well". Among the most interesting to us, wandering in Florence, are the two Andreas, one youthful and the other grown fatter than one likes and very different from the melancholy romantic figure in the Pitti; Verrocchio, by Lorenzo di Credi; Carlo Dolci, surprising by its good sense and humour; Raphael, angelic, wistful, and weak; Tintoretto, old and powerful; and Jacopo Bassano, old and simple. Among the moderns, Corot's portrait of himself is one of the most memorable, but Fantin Latour, Flandrin, Leon Bonnat, and Lenbach are all strong and modest; which one cannot say of our own Leighton. Among the later English heads Orchardson's is notable, but Mr. Sargent's is disappointing.

We now come to one of the most remarkable rooms in the gallery, where every picture is a gem; but since all are northern pictures, imported, I give no reproductions. This is the Sala di Van der Goes, so called from the great work here, the triptych, painted in 1474 to 1477 by Hugo van der Goes, who died in 1482, and was born at Ghent or Leyden about 1405. This painter, of whose genius there can be no question, is supposed to have been a pupil of the Van Eycks. Not much is known of him save that he painted at Bruges and Ghent and in 1476 entered a convent at Brussels where he was allowed to dine with distinguished strangers who came to see him and where he drank so much wine that his natural excitability turned to insanity. He seems, however, to have recovered, and if ever a picture showed few signs of a deranged or inflamed mind it is this, which was painted for the agent of the Medici bank at Bruges, Tommaso Portinari, who presented it to the Hospital of S. Maria Nuova in his native city of Florence, which had been founded by his ancestor Folco, the father of Dante's Beatrice. The left panel shows Tommaso praying with his two sons Antonio and Pigallo, the right his wife Maria Portinari and their adorably quaint little daughter with her charming head-dress and costume. The flowers in the centre panel are among the most beautiful things in any Florentine picture: not wild and wayward like Luca Signorelli's, but most exquisitely done: irises, red lilies, columbines and dark red clove pinks–

all unexpected and all very unlikely to be in such a wintry landscape at all. On the ground are violets. The whole work is grave, austere, cool, and as different as can be from the Tuscan spirit; yet it is said to have had a deep influence on the painters of the time and must have drawn throngs to the Hospital to see it.

The other Flemish and German pictures in the room are all remarkable and all warmer in tone. No. 906, an unknown work, is perhaps the finest: a Crucifixion, which might have borrowed its richness from the Carpaccio, we saw in the Venetian room. There is a fine Adoration of the Magi, by Gerard David (1460-1523); an unknown portrait of Pierantonio Baroncelli and his wife, with a lovely landscape; a jewel of paint by Hans Memling (1425-1492)–No. 703–the Madonna Enthroned; a masterpiece of drawing by Dürer, "Calvary"; an austere and poignant Transportation of Christ to the Sepulchre, by Roger van der Weyden (1400-1464); and several very beautiful portraits by Memling, notably Nos. 769 and 780 with their lovely evening light. Memling, indeed, I never liked better than here. Other fine pictures are a Spanish prince by Lucas van Leyden; an old Dutch scholar by an artist unknown, No. 784; and a young husband and wife by Joost van Cleef the Elder, and a Breughel the Elder, like an old Crome–a beauty–No. 928. The room is interesting both for itself and also as showing how the Flemish brushes were working at the time that so many of the great Italians were engaged on similar themes.

After the cool, self-contained, scientific work of these northerners it is a change to enter the Sala di Rubens and find that luxuriant giant–their compatriot, but how different!–once more. In the Uffizi, Rubens seems more foreign, far, than any one, so fleshly pagan is he. In Antwerp Cathedral his "Descent from the Cross," although its bravura is, as always with him, more noticeable than its piety, might be called a religious picture, but I doubt if even that would seem so here. At any rate his Uffizi works are all secular, while his "Holy Family" in the Pitti is merely domestic and robust. His Florentine masterpieces are the two Henri IV pictures in this room, "Henri IV at

Ivry," magnificent if not war, and "Henri's entry into Paris after Ivry," with its confusing muddle of naked warriors and spears. Only Rubens could have painted these spirited, impossible, glorious things, which for all their greatness send one's thoughts back longingly to the portrait of his wife, in the Tribuna, while No. 216–the Bacchanale–is so coarse as almost to send one's feet there too.

Looking round the room, after Rubens has been dismissed, it is too evident that the best of the Uffizi collection is behind us. There are interesting portraits here, but biographically rather than artistically. Here are one or two fine Sustermans' (1597-1681), that imported painter whom we shall find in such rare form at the Pitti. Here, for example, is Ferdinand II, who did so much for the Uffizi and so little for Galileo; and his cousin and wife Vittoria della Rovere, daughter of Claudia de' Medici (whose portrait, No. 763, is on the easel), and Federigo della Rovere, Duke of Urbino. This silly, plump lady had been married at the age of fourteen, and she brought her husband a little money and many pictures from Urbino, notably those delightful portraits of an earlier Duke and Duchess of Urbino by Piero della Francesca, and also the two Titian "Venuses" in the Tribuna. Ferdinand II and his Grand Duchess were on bad terms for most of their lives, and she behaved foolishly, and brought up her son Cosimo III foolishly, and altogether was a misfortune to Florence. Sustermans the painter she held in the highest esteem, and in return he painted her not only as herself but in various unlikely characters, among them a Vestal Virgin and even the Madonna.

Here also is No. 196, Van Dyck's portrait of Margherita of Lorraine, whose daughter became Cosimo III's wife–a mischievous, weak face but magnificently painted; and No. 1536, a vividly-painted elderly widow by Jordaens (1593-1678); and on each side of the outrageous Rubens a distinguished Dutch gentleman and lady by the placid, refined Mierevelt.

The two priceless rooms devoted to Iscrizioni come next, but we will finish the pictures first and therefore pass on to the Sala di Baroccio. Federigo Baroccio (1528-1612) is one of the later painters for whom I, at any rate, cannot feel any enthusiasm. His position in the Uffizi is due rather to the circumstance that he was a protégé of the Cardinal della Rovere at Rome, whose collection came here, than to his genius. This room again is of interest rather historically than artistically. Here, for example, are some good Medici portraits by Bronzino, among them the famous Eleanora of Toledo, wife of Cosimo I, in a rich brocade (in which she was buried), with the little staring Ferdinand I beside her. Eleanora, as we saw in chapter V. was the first mistress of the Pitti palace, and the lady who so disliked Cellini and got him into such trouble through his lying tongue. Bronzino's little Maria de' Medici–No. 1164–is more pleasing, for the other picture has a sinister air. This child, the first-born of Cosimo I and Eleanora, died when only sixteen. Baroccio has a fine portrait–Francesco Maria II, last Duke of Urbino, and the grandfather of the Vittoria della Rovere whom we saw in the Sala di Rubens. Here also is a portrait of Lorenzo the Magnificent by Vasari, but it is of small value since Vasari was not born till after Lorenzo's death. The Galileo by Sustermans–No. 163–on the contrary would be from life; and after the Tribuna portrait of Rubens' first wife it is interesting to find here his pleasant portrait of Helen Fourment, his second. To my eyes two of the most attractive pictures in the room are the Young Sculptor–No. 1266–by Bronzino, and the version of Leonardo's S. Anne at the Louvre by Andrea Salaino of Milan (1483?-1520?). I like also the hints of tenderness of Bernardino Luini which break through the hardness of the Aurelio Luini picture–No. 204. For the rest there are some sickly Guido Renis and Carlo Dolcis and a sentimental Guercino.

But the most popular works–on Sundays–are the two Gerard Honthorsts, and not without reason, for they are dramatic and bold and vivid, and there is a Baby in each that goes straight to the maternal heart. No. 157 is perhaps the more satisfying, but I have more reason to remember the larger one–the Adoration of the Shepherds–for I watched a copyist produce a most remarkable replica of it in something under a week, on the same scale. He was a short, swarthy man with a neck like a bull's, and he carried the task off with astonishing brio, never drawing a line, finishing each part as he came to it, and talking to a friend or an official the whole time. Somehow one felt him to be precisely the type of copyist that Gherardo della Notte ought to have. This painter was born at Utrecht in 1590 but went early to Italy, and settling in Rome devoted himself to mastering the methods of Amerighi, better known as Caravaggio (1569-1609), who specialized in strong contrasts of light and shade. After learning all he could in Rome, Honthorst returned to Holland and made much money and fame, for his hand was swift and sure. Charles I engaged him to decorate Whitehall. He died in 1656. These two Honthorsts are, as I say, the most popular of the pictures on Sunday, when the Uffizi is free; but their supremacy is challenged by the five inlaid tables, one of which, chiefly in lapis lazuli, must be the bluest thing on earth.

Passing for the present the Sala di Niobe, we come to the Sala di Giovanni di San Giovanni, which is given to a second-rate painter who was born in 1599 and died in 1636. His best work is a fresco at the Badia of Fiesole. Here he has some theatrical things, including one picture which sends English ladies out blushing. Here also are some Lelys, including "Nelly Gwynn". Next are two rooms, one leading from the other, given to German and Flemish pictures and to miniatures, both of which are interesting. In the first are more Dürers, and that alone would make it a desirable resort. Here is a "Virgin and Child"–No. 851–very naive and homely, and the beautiful portrait of his father–No. 766—a symphony of brown and green. Less attractive works from the same hand are the "Apostle Philip"–No. 777–and "S. Giacomo Maggiore," an old man very coarsely painted by comparison with the artist's father. Here also is a very beautiful portrait of Richard Southwell, by Holbein, with the peacock-green background that we know so well and always rejoice to see; a typical candle-light Schalcken, No. 800; several golden Poelenburghs; an anonymous portrait of Virgilius von Hytta of Zuicham, No. 784; a clever smiling lady by Sustermans, No. 709; the Signora Puliciani and her husband, No. 699; a rather crudely coloured Rubens–"Venus and Adonis"–No. 812; the same artist's "Three Graces," in monochrome, very naked; and some quaint portraits by Lucas Cranach.

But no doubt to many persons the most enchaining picture here is the Medusa's head, which used to be called a Leonardo and quite satisfied Ruskin of its genuineness, but is now attributed to the Flemish school. The head, at any rate, would seem to be very similar to that of which Vasari speaks, painted by Leonardo for a peasant, but retained by his father. Time has dealt hardly with the paint, and one has to study minutely before Medusa's horrors are visible. Whether Leonardo's or not, it is not uninteresting to read how the picture affected Shelley when he saw it here in 1819:–

... Its Horror and its Beauty are divine. Upon its lips and eyelids seem to lie Loveliness like a shadow, from which shine, Fiery and lurid, struggling underneath, The agonies of anguish and of death.

The little room leading from this one should be neglected by no one interested in Medicean history, for most of the family is here, in miniature, by Bronzino's hand. Here also are miniatures by other great painters, such as Pourbus, Guido Reni, Bassano, Clouet, Holbein. Look particularly at No. 3382, a woman with brown hair, in purple–a most fascinating little picture. The Ignota in No. 3348 might easily be Henrietta Maria, wife of Charles I of England. The other exhibits are copies in miniature of famous pictures, notable among them a Raphael No. 3386 and a Breughel–No. 3445–while No. 3341, the robing of a monk, is worth attention.

We come now to the last pictures of the collection–in three little rooms at the end, near the bronze sleeping Cupid. Those in the first room were being rearranged when I was last here; the others contain Dutch works notable for a few masterpieces. There are too many Poelenburghs, but the taste shown as a whole is good. Perhaps to the English enthusiast for painting the fine landscape by Hercules Seghers will, in view of the recent agitation over Lord Lansdowne's Rembrandt, "The Mill,"–ascribed in some quarters to Seghers–be the most interesting picture of all. It is a sombre, powerful scene of rugged coast which any artist would have been proud to sign; but it in no way recalls "The Mill's" serene strength. Among the best of its companions are a very good Terburg, a very good Metsu, and an extremely beautiful Ruysdael.

And so we are at the end of the pictures–but only to return again and again–and are not unwilling to fall into the trap of the official who sits here, and allow him to unlock the door behind the Laocöon group and enjoy what he recommends as a "bella vista" from the open space, which turns out to be the roof of the Loggia de' Lanzi. From this high point one may see much of Florence and its mountains, while, on looking down, over the coping, one finds the busy Piazza della Signoria below, with all its cabs and wayfarers.

Returning to the gallery, we come quickly on the right to the first of the neglected statuary rooms, the beautiful Sala di Niobe, which contains some interesting Medicean and other tapestries, and the sixteen statues of Niobe and her children from the Temple of Apollo, which the Cardinal Ferdinand de' Medici acquired, and which were for many years at the Villa Medici at Rome. A suggested reconstruction of the group will be found by the door. I cannot pretend to a deep interest in the figures, but I like to be in the room. The famous Medicean vase is in the middle of it. Sculpture more ingratiating is close by, in the two rooms given to Iscrizioni: a collection of priceless antiques which are not only beautiful but peculiarly interesting in that they can be compared with the work of Donatello, Verrocchio, and other of the Renaissance sculptors. For in such a case comparisons are anything but odious and become fascinating. In the first room there is, for example, a Mercury, isolated on the left, in marble, who is a blood relation of Donatello's bronze David in the Bargello; and certain reliefs of merry children, on the right, low down, as one approaches the second room, are cousins of the same sculptor's cantoria romps. Not that Donatello ever reproduced the antique spirit as Michelangelo nearly did in his Bacchus, and Sansovino absolutely did in his Bacchus, both at the Bargello: Donatello was of his time, and the spirit of his time animates his creations, but he had studied the Greek art in Rome and profited by his lessons, and his evenly-balanced humane mind had a warm corner for pagan joyfulness. Among other statues in this first room is a Sacerdotessa, wearing a marble robe with long folds, whose hands can be seen through the drapery. Opposite the door are Bacchus and Ampelos, superbly pagan, while a sleeping Cupid is most lovely. Among the various fine heads is one of Cicero, of an Unknown–No. 377–and of Homer in bronze (called by the photographers Aristophanes). But each thing in turn is almost the best. The trouble is that the Uffizi is so vast, and the Renaissance seems to be so eminently the only proper study of mankind when one is here, that to attune oneself to the enjoyment of antique sculpture needs a special effort which not all are ready to make.

In the centre of the next room is the punctual Hermaphrodite without which no large Continental gallery is complete. But more worthy of attention is the torso of a faun on the left, on a revolving pedestal which (unlike those in the Bargello, as we shall discover) really does revolve and enables you to admire the perfect back. There is also a torso in basalt or porphyry which one should study from all points, and on the walls some wonderful portions of a frieze from the Ara Pacis, erected in Rome, B.C. 139, with wonderful figures of men, women, and children on it. Among the heads is a colossal Alexander, very fine indeed, a beautiful Antoninus, a benign and silly Roman lady in whose existence one can quite believe, and a melancholy Seneca. Look also at Nos. 330 and 332, on the wall: 330, a charming genius, carrying one of Jove's thunderbolts; and 332, a boy who is sheer Luca della Robbia centuries before his birth.

I ought to add that, in addition to the various salons in the Uffizi, the long corridors are hung with pictures too, in chronological order, the earliest of all being to the right of the entrance door, and in the corridors there is also some admirable statuary. But the pictures here, although not the equals of those in the rooms, receive far too little attention, while the sculpture receives even less, whether the beutiful full-length athletes or the reliefs on the cisterns, several of which have riotous Dionysian processions. On the stairs, too, are some very beautiful works; while at the top, in the turnstile room, is the original of the boar which Tacca copied in bronze for the Mercato Nuovo, and just outside it are the Medici who were chiefly concerned with the formation of the collection. On the first landing, nearest the ground, is a very beautiful and youthful Bacchus. The ceilings of the Uffizi rooms and corridors also are painted, thoughtfully and dexterously, in the Pompeian manner; but there are limits to the receptive capacity of travellers' eyes, and I must plead guilty to consistently neglecting them.

CHAPTER XII

"Aërial Fiesole"

Andrea del Sarto–Fiesole sights–The Villa Palmieri and the "Decameron"–Botticini's picture in the National Gallery–S. Francesco–The Roman amphitheatre–The Etruscan museum–A sculptor's walk–The Badia di Fiesole–Brunelleschi again–Giovanni di San Giovanni.

After all these pictures, how about a little climbing? From so many windows in Florence, along so many streets, from so many loggias and towers, and perhaps, above all, from the Piazzale di Michelangelo, Fiesole is to be seen on her hill, with the beautiful campanile of her church in the dip between the two eminences, that very soon one comes to feel that this surely is the promised land. Florence lies so low, and the delectable mountain is so near and so alluring. But I am not sure that to dream of Fiesole as desirable, and to murmur its beautiful syllables, is not best.

Let me sit Here by the window with your hand in mine, And look a half-hour forth on Fiesole

–that was Andrea's way and not an unwise one. For Fiesole at nearer view can easily disappoint. It is beautifully set on its hill and it has a fascinating past; but the journey thither on foot is very wearisome, by the electric tram vexatious and noisy, and in a horse-drawn carriage expensive and cruel; and when you are there you become once more a tourist without alleviation and are pestered by beggars, and by nice little girls who ought to know better, whose peculiar importunacy it is to thrust flowers into the hand or buttonhole without any denial. What should have been a mountain retreat from the city has become a kind of Devil's Dyke. But if one is resolute, and, defying all, walks up to the little monastery of S. Francesco at the very top of the hill, one may rest almost undisturbed, with Florence in the valley below, and gardens and vineyards undulating beneath, and a monk or two ascending or descending the steps, and three or four picture-postcard hawkers gambling in a corner, and lizards on the wall. Here it is good to be in the late afternoon, when the light is mellowing; and if you want tea there is a little loggia a few yards down this narrow steep path where it may be found. How many beautiful villas in which one could be happy sunning oneself among the lizards lie between this point and Florence! Who, sitting here, can fail to think that?

In walking to Fiesole one follows the high walls of the Villa Palmieri, which is now very private American property, but is famous for ever as the first refuge of Boccaccio's seven young women and three young men when they fled from plague-stricken Florence in 1348 and told tales for ten halcyon days. It is now generally agreed that if Boccaccio had any particular house in his mind it was this. It used to be thought that the Villa Poggio Gherardo, Mrs. Ross's beautiful home on the way to Settignano, was the first refuge, and the Villa Palmieri the second, but the latest researches have it that the Palmieri was the first and the Podere della Fonte, or Villa di Boccaccio, as it is called, near Camerata, a little village below S. Domenico, the other. The Villa Palmieri has another and somewhat different historical association, for it was there that Queen Victoria resided for a while in 1888. But the most interesting thing of all about it is the circumstance that it was the home of Matteo Palmieri, the poet, and Botticelli's friend and fellow-speculator on the riddle of life. Palmieri was the author of a remarkable poem called "La Citta della Vita" (The City of Life) which developed a scheme of theology that had many attractions to Botticelli's curious mind. The poem was banned by Rome, although not until after its author's death. In our National Gallery is a picture which used to be considered Botticelli's–No. 1126, "The Assumption of the Virgin"–especially as it is mentioned with some particularity by Vasari, together with the circumstance that the poet and painter devised it in collaboration, in which the poem is translated into pigment. As to the theology, I say nothing, nor as to its new ascription to Botticini; but the picture has a greater interest for us in that it contains a view of Florence with its wall of towers around it in about 1475. The exact spot where the painter sat has been identified by Miss Stokes in "Six Months in the Apennines". On the left immediately below the painter's vantage-ground is the Mugnone, with a bridge over it. On the bank in front is the Villa Palmieri, and on the picture's extreme left is the Badia of Fiesole.

On leaving S. Domenico, if still bent on walking, one should keep straight on and not follow the tram lines to the right. This is the old and terribly steep road which Lorenzo the Magnificent and his friends Politian and Pico della Mirandola had to travel whenever they visited the Medici villa, just under Fiesole, with its drive lined with cypresses. Here must have been great talk and much conviviality. It is now called the Villa McCalmont.

Once at Fiesole, by whatever means you reach it, do not neglect to climb the monastery steps to the very top. It is a day of climbing, and a hundred or more steps either way mean nothing now. For here is a gentle little church with swift, silent monks in it, and a few flowers in bowls, and a religious picture by that strange Piero di Cosimo whose heart was with the gods in exile; and the view of Monte Ceceri, on the other side of Fiesole, seen through the cypresses here, which could not be better in disposition had Benozzo Gozzoli himself arranged them, is very striking and memorable.

Fiesole's darling son is Mino the sculptor–the "Raphael of the chisel"–whose radiant Madonnas and children and delicate tombs may be seen here and there all over Florence. The piazza is named after him; he is celebrated on a marble slab outside the museum, where all the famous names of the vicinity may be read too; and in the church is one of his most charming groups and finest heads. They are in a little chapel on the right of the choir. The head is that of Bishop Salutati, humorous, wise, and benign, and the group represents the adoration of a merry little Christ by a merry little S. John and others. As for the church itself, it is severe and cool, with such stone columns in it as must last for ever.

But the main interest of Fiesole to most people is not the cypress-covered hill of S. Francesco; not the view from the summit; not the straw mementoes; not the Mino relief in the church; but the Roman arena. The excavators have made of this a very complete place. One can stand at the top of the steps and reconstruct it all–the audience, the performance, the performers. A very little time spent on building would be needed to restore the amphitheatre to its original form. Beyond it are baths, and in a hollow the remains of a temple with the altar where it ever was; and then one walks a little farther and is on the ancient Etruscan wall, built when Fiesole was an Etruscan fortified hill city. So do the centuries fall away here! But everywhere, among the ancient Roman stones so massive and exact, and the Etruscan stones, are the wild flowers which Luca Signorelli painted in that picture in the Uffizi which I love so much.

After the amphitheatre one visits the Museum–with the same ticket–a little building filled with trophies of the spade. There is nothing very wonderful–nothing to compare with the treasures of the Archaeological Museum in Florence–but it is well worth a visit.

On leaving the Museum on the last occasion that I was there–in April–I walked to Settignano. The road for a while is between houses, for Fiesole stretches a long way farther than one suspects, very high, looking over the valley of the Mugnone; and then after a period between pine trees and grape-hyacinths one turns to the right and begins to descend. Until Poggio del Castello, a noble villa, on an isolated eminence, the descent is very gradual, with views of Florence round the shoulder of Monte Ceceri; but afterwards the road winds, to ease the fall, and the wayfarer turns off into the woods and tumbles down the hill by a dry water-course, amid crags and stones, to the beginnings of civilization again, at the Via di Desiderio da Settignano, a sculptor who stands to his native town in precisely the same relation as Mino to his.

Settignano is a mere village, with villas all about it, and the thing to remember there is not only that Desiderio was born there but that Michelangelo's foster-mother was the wife of a local stone-cutter–stone-cutting at that time being the staple industry. On the way back to Florence in the tram, one passes on the right a gateway surmounted by statues of the poets, the Villa Poggio Gherardo, of which I have spoken earlier in the chapter. There is no villa with a nobler mien than this.

That is one walk from Fiesole. Another is even more a sculptors' way: for it would include Maiano too, where Benedetto was born. The road is by way of the tram lines to that acute angle just below Fiesole when they turn back to S. Domenico, and so straight on down the hill.

But if one is returning to Florence direct after leaving Fiesole it is well to walk down the precipitous paths to S. Domenico, and before again taking the tram visit the Badia overlooking the valley of the Mugnone. This is done by turning to the right just opposite the church of S. Domenico, which has little interest structurally but is famous as being the chapel of the monastery where Fra Angelico was once a monk. The Badia (Abbey) di Fiesole, as it now is, was built on the site of an older monastery, by Cosimo Pater. Here Marsilio Ficino's Platonic Academy used to meet, in the loggia and in the little temple which one gains from the cloisters, and here Pico della Mirandola composed his curious gloss on Genesis.

The dilapidated marble façade of the church and its rugged stone-work are exceedingly ancient–dating in fact from the eleventh century; the new building is by Brunelleschi and to my mind is one of his most beautiful works, its lovely proportions and cool, unfretted white spaces communicating even more pleasure than the Pazzi chapel itself. The decoration has been kept simple and severe, and the colour is just the grey pietra serena of Fiesole, of which the lovely arches are made, all most exquisitely chiselled, and the pure white of the walls and ceilings. This church was a favourite with the Medici, and the youthful Giovanni, the son of Lorenzo the Magnificent, received his cardinal's hat here in 1492, at the age of sixteen. He afterwards became Pope Leo X. How many of the boys, now in the school–for the monastery has become a Jesuit school–will, one wonders, rise to similar eminence.

In the beautiful cloisters we have the same colour scheme as in the church, and here again Brunelleschi's miraculous genius for proportion is to be found. Here and there are foliations and other exquisite tracery by pupils of Desiderio da Settignano. The refectory has a high-spirited fresco by that artist whose room in the Uffizi is so carefully avoided by discreet chaperons–Giovanni di San Giovanni–representing Christ eating at a table, his ministrants being a crowd of little roguish angels and cherubim, one of whom (on the right) is in despair at having broken a plate. In the entrance lobby is a lavabo by Mino da Fiesole, with two little boys of the whitest and softest marble on it, which is worth study.

And now we will return to the heart of Florence once more.

CHAPTER XIII

THE Badia and Dante

Filippino Lippi–Buffalmacco–Mino da Fiesole–The Dante quarter–Dante and Beatrice–Monna Tessa–Gemma Donati–Dante in exile–Dante memorials in Florence–The Torre della Castagna–The Borgo degli Albizzi and the old palaces–S. Ambrogio–Mino's tabernacle–Wayside masterpieces–S. Egidio.

Opposite the Bargello is a church with a very beautiful doorway designed by Benedetto da Rovezzano. This church is known as the Badia, and its delicate spire is a joy in the landscape from every point of vantage. The Badia is very ancient, but the restorers have been busy and little of Arnolfo's thirteenth-century work is left. It is chiefly famous now for its Filippino Lippi and two tombs by Mino da Fiesole, but historically it is interesting as being the burial-place of the chief Florentine families in the Middle Ages and as being the scene of Boccaccio's lectures on Dante in 1373. The Filippino altar-piece, which represents S. Bernard's Vision of the Virgin (a subject we shall see treated very beautifully by Fra Bartolommeo at the Accademia) is one of the most perfect and charming pictures by this artist: very grave and real and sweet, and the saint's hands exquisitely painted. The figure praying in the right-hand corner is the patron, Piero di Francesco del Pugliese, who commissioned this picture for the church of La Campora, outside the Porta Romana, where it was honoured until 1529, when Clement VII's troops advancing, it was brought here for safety and has here remained.

Close by–in the same chapel–is a little door which the sacristan will open, disclosing a portion of Arnolfo's building with perishing frescoes which are attributed to Buffalmacco, an artist as to whose reality much scepticism prevails. They are not in themselves of much interest, although the sacristan's eagerness should not be discouraged; but Buffalmacco being Boccaccio's, Sacchetti's, Vasari's (and, later, Anatole France's) amusing hero, it is pleasant to look at his work and think of his freakishness. Buffalmacco (if he ever existed) was one of the earlier painters, flourishing between 1311 and 1350, and was a pupil of Andrea Tafi. This simple man he plagued very divertingly, once frightening him clean out of his house by fixing little lighted candles to the backs of beetles and steering them into Tafi's bedroom at night. Tafi was terrified, but on being told by Buffalmacco (who was a lazy rascal) that these devils were merely showing their objection to early rising, he became calm again, and agreed to lie in bed to a reasonable hour. Cupidity, however, conquering, he again ordered his pupil to be up betimes, when the beetles again re-appeared and continued to do so until the order was revoked.

The sculptor Mino da Fiesole, whom we shall shortly see again, at the Bargello, in portrait busts and Madonna reliefs, is at his best here, in the superb monument to Count Ugo, who founded, with his mother, the Benedictine Abbey of which the Badia is the relic. Here all Mino's sweet thoughts, gaiety and charm are apparent, together with the perfection of radiant workmanship. The quiet dignity of the recumbent figure is no less masterly than the group above it. Note the impulsive urgency of the splendid Charity, with her two babies, and the quiet beauty of the Madonna and Child above all, while the proportions and delicate patterns of the tomb as a whole still remain to excite one's pleasure and admiration. We shall see many tombs in Florence–few not beautiful–but none more joyously accomplished than this. The tomb of Carlo Marsuppini in S. Croce by Desiderio da Settignano, which awaits us, was undoubtedly the parent of the Ugo, Mino following his master very closely; but his charm was his own. According to Vasari, the Ugo tomb was considered to be Mino's finest achievement, and he deliberately made the Madonna and Child as like the types of his beloved Desiderio as he could. It was finished in 1481, and Mino died in 1484, from a chill following over-exertion in moving heavy stones. Mino also has here a monument to Bernardo Giugni, a famous gonfalonier in the time of Cosimo de' Medici, marked by the same distinction, but not quite so memorable. The Ugo is his masterpiece.

The carved wooden ceiling, which is a very wonderful piece of work and of the deepest and most glorious hue, should not be forgotten; but nothing is easier than to overlook ceilings.

The cloisters are small, but they atone for that–if it is a fault–by having a loggia. From the loggia the top of the noble tower of the Palazzo Vecchio is seen to perfection. Upon the upper walls is a series of frescoes illustrating the life of S. Benedict which must have been very gay and spirited once but are now faded.

The Badia may be said to be the heart of the Dante quarter. Dante must often have been in the church before it was restored as we now see it, and a quotation from the "Divine Comedy" is on its façade. The Via Dante and the Piazza Donati are close by, and in the Via Dante are many reminders of the poet besides his alleged birthplace. Elsewhere in the city we find incised quotations from his poem; but the Baptistery–his "beautiful San Giovanni"–is the only building in the city proper now remaining which Dante would feel at home in could he return to it, and where we can feel assured of sharing his presence. The same pavement is there on which his feet once stood, and on the same mosaic of Christ above the altar would his eyes have fallen. When Dante was exiled in 1302 the cathedral had been in progress only for six or eight years; but it is known that he took the deepest interest in its construction, and we have seen the stone marking the place where he sat, watching the builders. The façade of the Badia of Fiesole and the church of S. Miniato can also remember Dante; no others.

Here, however, we are on that ground which is richest in personal associations with him and his, for in spite of re-building and certain modern changes the air is heavy with antiquity in these narrow streets and passages where the poet had his childhood and youth. The son of a lawyer named Alighieri, Dante was born in 1265, but whether or not in this Casa Dante is an open question, and it was in the Baptistery that he received the name of Durante, afterwards abbreviated to Dante–Durante meaning enduring, and Dante giving. Those who have read the "Vita Nuova," either in the original or in Rossetti's translation, may be surprised to learn that the boy was only nine when he first met his Beatrice, who was seven, and for ever passed into bondage to her. Who Beatrice was is again a mystery, but it has been agreed to consider her in real life a daughter of Folco Portinari, a wealthy Florentine and the founder of the hospital of S. Maria Nuova, one of whose descendants commissioned Hugo van der Goes to paint the great triptych in the Uffizi. Folco's tomb is in S. Egidio, the hospital church, while in the passage to the cloisters is a stone figure of Monna Tessa (of whom we are about to see a coloured bust in the Bargello), who was not only Beatrice's nurse (if Beatrice were truly of the Portinari) but the instigator, it is said, of Folco's deed of charity.

Of Dante's rapt adoration of his lady, the "Vita Nuova" tells. According to that strangest monument of devotion it was not until another nine years had passed that he had speech of her; and then Beatrice, meeting him in the street, saluted him as she passed him with such ineffable courtesy and grace that he was lifted into a seventh heaven of devotion and set upon the writing of his book. The two seem to have had no closer intercourse: Beatrice shone distantly like a star and her lover worshipped her with increasing loyalty and fervour, overlaying the idea of her, as one might say, with gold and radiance, very much as we shall see Fra Angelico adding glory to the Madonna and Saints in his pictures, and with a similar intensity of ecstasy. Then one day Beatrice married, and not long afterwards, being always very fragile, she died, at the age of twenty-three. The fact that she was no longer on earth hardly affected her poet, whose worship of her had always so little of a physical character; and she continued to dominate his thoughts.

In 1293, however, Dante married, one Gemma Donati of the powerful Guelph family of that name, of which Corso Donati was the turbulent head; and by her he had many children. For Gemma, however, he seems to have had no affection; and when in 1301 he left Florence, never to return, he left his wife for ever too. In 1289 Dante had been present at the battle of Campaldino, fighting with the Guelphs against the Ghibellines, and on settling down in Florence and taking to politics it was as a Guelph, or rather as one of that branch of the Guelph party which had become White–the Bianchi–as opposed to the other party which was Black–the Neri. The feuds between these divisions took the place of those between the Guelphs and Ghibellines, since Florence was never happy without internal strife, and it cannot have added to Dante's home comfort that his wife was related to Corso Donati, who led the Neri and swaggered in his bullying way about the city with proprietary, intolerant airs that must have been infuriating to a man with Dante's stern sense of right and justice. It was Corso who brought about Dante's exile; but he himself survived only six years, and was then killed, by his own wish, on his way to execution, rather than be humiliated in the city in which he had swayed. Dante, whose genius devised a more lasting form of reprisal than any personal encounter could be, has depicted him in the "Purgatorio" as on the road to Hell.

But this is going too fast. In 1300, when Dante was thirty-five, he was sufficiently important to be made one of the six priors of the city, and in that capacity was called upon to quell a Neri and Bianchi disturbance. It is characteristic of him that he was a party to the banishment of the leaders of both factions, among whom was his closest friend, Guido Cavalcanti the poet, who was one of the Bianchi. Whether it was because of Guide's illness in his exile, or from what motive, we shall not know; but the sentence was lightened in the case of this Bianco, a circumstance which did not add to Dante's chances when the Neri, having plotted successfully with Charles of Valois, captured supreme power in Florence. This was in the year 1301, Dante being absent from that city on an embassy to Rome to obtain help for the Bianchi. He never came back; for the Neri plans succeeded; the Neri assumed control; and in January, 1302, he was formally fined and banished. The nominal charge against him was of misappropriating funds while a prior; but that was merely a matter of form. His real offence was in being one of the Bianchi, an enemy of the Neri, and a man of parts.

In the rest of Dante's life Florence had no part, except in his thoughts. How he viewed her the "Divine Comedy" tells us, and that he longed to return we also know. The chance was indeed once offered, but under the impossible condition that he should do public penance in the Baptistery for his offence. This he refused. He wandered here and there, and settled finally in Ravenna, where he died in 1321. The "Divine Comedy" anticipating printing by so many years–the invention did not reach Florence until 1471–Dante could not make much popular way as a poet before that time; but to his genius certain Florentines were earlier no strangers, not only by perusing MS. copies of his great work, which by its richness in Florentine allusions excited an interest apart altogether from that created by its beauty, but by public lectures on the poem, delivered in the churches by order of the Signoria. The first Dante professor to be appointed was Giovanni Boccaccio, the author of the "Decameron," who was born in 1313, eight years before Dante's death, and became an enthusiast upon the poet. The picture in the Duomo was placed there in 1465. Then came printing to Florence and Dante passed quickly into his countrymen's thoughts and language.

Michelangelo, who was born in time–1475–to enjoy in Lorenzo the Magnificent's house the new and precious advantage of printed books, became as a boy a profound student of the poet, and when later an appeal was made from Florence to the Pope to sanction the removal of Dante's bones to Florence, Michelangelo was among the signatories. But it was not done. His death-mask from Ravenna is in the Bargello: a few of his bones and their coffin are still in Ravenna, in the monastery of Classe, piously preserved in a room filled with Dante relics and literature; his tomb is elsewhere at Ravenna, a shrine visited by thousands every year.

Ever since has Dante's fame been growing, so that only the Bible has led to more literature; and to-day Florence is more proud of him than any of her sons, except perhaps Michelangelo. We have seen one or two reminders of him already; more are here where we stand. We have seen the picture in honour of him which the Republic set up in the cathedral; his head on a beautiful inlaid door in the Palazzo Vecchio, the building where his sentence of banishment was devised and carried, to be followed by death sentence thrice repeated (burning alive, to be exact); and we have seen the head-quarters of the Florentine Dante society in the guild house at Or San Michele. We have still to see his statue opposite S. Croce, another fresco head in S. Maria Novella, certain holograph relics at the library at S. Lorenzo, and his head again by his friend Giotto, in the Bargello, where he would have been confined while waiting for death had he been captured.

Dante's house has been rebuilt, very recently, and next to it is a newer building still, with a long inscription in Italian upon it, to the effect that the residence of Bella and Bellincione Alighieri stood hereabouts, and in that abode was Dante born. The Commune of Florence, it goes on to say, having secured possession of the site, "built this edifice on the remains of the ancestral house as fresh evidence of the public veneration of the divine poet". The Torre della Castagna, across the way, has an inscription in Italian, which may be translated thus: "This Tower, the so-called Tower of the Chestnut, is the solitary remnant of the head-quarters from which the Priors of the Arts governed Florence, before the power and glory of the Florentine Commune procured the erection of the Palace of the Signoria".

Few persons in the real city of Florence, it may be said confidently, live in a house built for them; but hereabouts none at all. In fact, it is the exception anywhere near the centre of the city to live in a house built less than three centuries ago. Palaces abound, cut up into offices, flats, rooms, and even cinema theatres. The telegraph office in the Via del Proconsolo is a palace commissioned by the Strozzi but never completed: hence its name, Non-finito; next it is the superb Palazzo Quaratesi, which Brunelleschi designed, now the head-quarters of a score of firms and an Ecclesiastical School whence sounds of sacred song continually emerge.

Since we have Mino da Fiesole in our minds and are on the subject of old palaces let us walk from the Dante quarter in a straight line from the Corso, that very busy street of small shops, across the Via del Proconsolo and down the Borgo degli Albizzi to S. Ambrogio, where Mino was buried. This Borgo is a street of palaces and an excellent one in which to reflect upon the strange habit which wealthy Florentines then indulged of setting their mansions within a few feet of those opposite. Houses–or rather fortresses–that must have cost fortunes and have been occupied by families of wealth and splendour were erected so close to their vis-à-vis that two carts could not pass abreast between them. Side by side contiguity one can understand, but not this other adjacence. Every ground floor window is barred like a gaol. Those bars tell us something of the perils of life in Florence in the great days of faction ambition; while the thickness of the walls and solidity of construction tell us something too of the integrity of the Florentine builders. These ancient palaces, one feels, whatever may happen to them, can never fall to ruin. Such stones as are placed one upon the other in the Pitti and the Strozzi and the Riccardi nothing can displace. It is an odd thought that several Florentine palaces and villas built before Columbus sailed for America are now occupied by rich Americans, some of them draw possibly much of their income from the manufacture of steel girders for sky-scrapers. These ancient streets with their stern and sombre palaces specially touched the imagination of Dickens when he was in Florence in 1844, but in his "Pictures from Italy" he gave the city only fugitive mention. The old prison, which then adjoined the Palazzo Vecchio, and in which the prisoners could be seen, also moved him.

The Borgo degli Albizzi, as I have said, is crowded with Palazzi. No. 24–and there is something very incongruous in palaces having numbers at all–is memorable in history as being one of the homes of the Pazzi family who organized the conspiracy against the Medici in 1478, as I have related in the second chapter, and failed so completely. Donatello designed the coat of arms here. The palace at No. 18 belonged to the Altoviti. No. 12 is the Palazzo Albizzi, the residence of one of the most powerful of the Florentine families, whose allies were all about them in this quarter, as it was wise to be.

As a change from picture galleries, I can think of nothing more delightful than to wander about these ancient streets, and, wherever a courtyard or garden shines, penetrate to it; stopping now and again to enjoy the vista, the red Duomo, or Giotto's tower, so often mounting into the sky at one end, or an indigo Apennine at the other. Standing in the middle of the Via Ricasoli, for example, one has sight of both.

At the Piazza S. Pietro we see one of the old towers of Florence, of which there were once so many, into which the women and children might retreat in times of great danger, and here too is a series of arches which fruit and vegetable shops make gay.

The next Piazza is that of S. Ambrogio. This church is interesting not only for doing its work in a poor quarter–one has the feeling at once that it is a right church in the right place–but as containing, as I have said, the grave of Mino da Fiesole: Mino de' Poppi detto da Fiesole, as the floor tablet has it. Over the altar of Mino's little chapel is a large tabernacle from his hand, in which the gayest little Boy gives the benediction, own brother to that one by Desiderio at S. Lorenzo. The tabernacle must be one of the master's finest works, and beneath it is a relief in which a priest pours something–perhaps the very blood of Christ which is kept here–from one chalice to another held by a kneeling woman, surrounded by other kneeling women, which is a marvel of flowing beauty and life. The lines of it are peculiarly lovely.

On the wall of the same little chapel is a fresco by Cosimo Rosselli which must once have been a delight, representing a procession of Corpus Christi–this chapel being dedicated to the miracle of the Sacrament–and it contains, according to Vasari, a speaking likeness of Pico della Mirandola. Other graves in the church are those of Cronaca, the architect of the Palazzo Vecchio's great Council Room, a friend of Savonarola and Rosselli's nephew by marriage; and Verrocchio, the sculptor, whose beautiful work we are now to see in the Bargello. It is said that Lorenzo di Credi also lies here, and Albertinelli, who gave up the brush for innkeeping.

Opposite the church, on a house at the corner of the Borgo S. Croce and the Via de' Macci, is a della Robbia saint–one of many such mural works of art in Florence. Thus, at the corner of the Via Cavour and the Via de' Pucci, opposite the Riccardi palace, is a beautiful Madonna and Child by Donatello. In the Via Zannetti, which leads out of the Via Cerretani, is a very pretty example by Mino, a few houses on the right. These are sculpture. And everywhere in the older streets you may see shrines built into the wall: there is even one in the prison, in the Via dell' Agnolo, once the convent of the Murate, where Catherine de' Medici was imprisoned as a girl; but many of them are covered with glass which has been allowed to become black.

A word or two on S. Egidio, the church of the great hospital of S. Maria Nuova, might round off this chapter, since it was Folco Portinari, Beatrice's father, who founded it. The hospital stands in a rather forlorn square a few steps from the Duomo, down the Via dell' Orivolo and then the first to the left; and it extends right through to the Via degli Alfani in cloisters and ramifications. The façade is in a state of decay, old frescoes peeling off it, but one picture has been enclosed for protection–a gay and busy scene of the consecration of the church by Pope Martin V. Within, it is a church of the poor, notable for its general florid comfort (comparatively) and Folco's gothic tomb. In the chancel is a pretty little tabernacle by Mino, which used to have a bronze door by Ghiberti, but has it no longer, and a very fine della Robbia Madonna and Child, probably by Andrea. Behind a grille, upstairs, sit the hospital nurses. In the adjoining cloisters–one of the high roads to the hospital proper–is the ancient statue of old Monna Tessa, Beatrice's nurse, and, in a niche, a pretty symbolical painting of Charity by that curious painter Giovanni di San Giovanni. It was in the hospital that the famous Van der Goes triptych used to hang.

A tablet on a house opposite S. Egidio, a little to the right, states that it was there that Ghiberti made the Baptistery gates which Michelangelo considered fit to be the portals of Paradise.

CHAPTER XIV

THE Bargello

Plastic art–Blood-soaked stones–The faithful artists–Michelangelo–Italian custodians–The famous Davids–Michelangelo's tondo–Brutus–Benedetto da Rovezzano–Donatello's life-work–The S. George–Verrocchio–Ghiberti and Brunelleschi and the Baptistery doors–Benvenuto Cellini–John of Bologna–Antonio Pollaiuolo–Verrocchio again–Mino da Fiesole–The Florentine wealth of sculpture–Beautiful ladies–The della Robbias–South Kensington and the Louvre.

Before my last visit but one to Florence, plastic art was less attractive to me than pictorial art. But now I am not sure. At any rate when, here in England, I think of Florence, as so often I do, I find myself visiting in imagination the Bargello before the Uffizi. Pictures in any number can bewilder and dazzle as much as they delight. The eye tires. And so, it is true, can a multiplicity of antique statuary such as one finds at the Vatican or at the Louvre; but a small collection of Renaissance work, so soft and human, as at the Bargello, is not only joy-giving but refreshing too. The soft contours soothe as well as enrapture the eye: the tenderness of the Madonnas, the gentleness of the Florentine ladies and youths, as Verrocchio and Mino da Fiesole, Donatello, and Pollaiuolo moulded them, calm one where the perfection of Phidias and Praxiteles excites. Hence the very special charm of the Bargello, whose plastic treasures are comparatively few and picked, as against the heaped profusion of paint in the Uffizi and the Pitti. It pairs off rather with the Accademia, and has this further point in common with that choicest of galleries, that Michelangelo's chisel is represented in both.

The Bargello is at the corner of the Via Ghibellina in the narrow Via del Proconsolo–so narrow that if you take one step off the pavement a tram may easily sweep you into eternity; so narrow also that the real dignity of the Bargello is never to be properly seen, and one thinks of it rather for its inner court and staircase and its strong tower than for its massive façades. Its history is soaked in blood. It was built in the middle of the thirteenth century as the residence of the chief magistrate of the city, the Capitano del popolo, or Podestà, first appointed soon after the return of the Guelphs in 1251, and it so remained, with such natural Florentine vicissitudes as destruction by mobs and fire, for four hundred years, when, in 1574, it was converted into a prison and place of execution and the head-quarters of the police, and changed its name from the Palazzo del Podestà to that by which it is now known, so called after the Bargello, or chief of the police.

It is indeed fortunate that no rioters succeeded in obliterating Giotto's fresco in the Bargello chapel, which he painted probably in 1300, when his friend Dante was a Prior of the city. Giotto introduced the portrait of Dante which has drawn so many people to this little room, together with portraits of Corso Donati, and Brunetto Latini, Dante's tutor. Whitewash covered it for two centuries. Dante's head has been restored.

It was in 1857 that the Bargello was again converted, this time to its present gracious office of preserving the very flower of Renaissance plastic art.

Passing through the entrance hall, which has a remarkable collection of Medicean armour and weapons, and in which (I have read but not seen) is an oubliette under one of the great pillars, the famous court is gained and the famous staircase. Of this court what can I say? Its quality is not to be communicated in words; and even the photographs of it that are sold have to be made from pictures, which the assiduous Signor Giuliani, among others, is always so faithfully painting, stone for stone. One forgets all the horrors that once were enacted here–the execution of honourable Florentine patriots whose only offence was that in their service of this proud and beautiful city they differed from those in power; one thinks only of the soft light on the immemorial walls, the sturdy graceful columns, the carved escutcheons, the resolute steps, the spaciousness and stern calm of it all.

In the colonnade are a number of statues, the most famous of which is perhaps the "Dying Adonis" which Baedeker gives to Michelangelo but the curator to Vincenzo di Rossi; an ascription that would annoy Michelangelo exceedingly, if it were a mistake, since Rossi was a pupil of his enemy, the absurd Bandinelli. Mr. W.G. Waters, in his "Italian Sculptors," considers not only that Michelangelo was the sculptor, but that the work was intended to form part of the tomb of Pope Julius. In the second room opposite the main entrance across the courtyard, we come however to Michelangelo authentic and supreme, for here are his small David, his Brutus, his Bacchus, and a tondo of the Madonna and Child.

According to Baedeker the Bacchus and the David revolve. Certainly they are on revolving stands, but to say that they revolve is to disregard utterly the character of the Italian official. A catch holds each in its place, and any effort to release this or to induce the custodian to release it is equally futile. "Chiuso" (closed), he replies, and that is final. Useless to explain that the backs of statues can be beautiful as the front; that one of the triumphs of great statuary is its equal perfection from every point; that the revolving stand was not made for a joke but for a serious purpose. "Chiuso," he replies. The museum custodians of Italy are either like this–jaded figures of apathy–or they are enthusiasts. To each enthusiast there are ninety-nine of the other, who either sit in a kind of stupor and watch you with sullen suspicion, or clear their throats as no gentleman should. The result is that when one meets the enthusiasts one remembers them. There is a little dark fellow in the Brera at Milan whose zeal in displaying the merits of Mantegna's foreshortened Christ is as unforgettable as a striking piece of character-acting in a theatre. There is a more reserved but hardly less appreciative official in the Accademia at Bologna with a genuine if incommunicable passion for Guido Reni. And, lastly, there is Alfred Branconi, at S. Croce, with his continual and rapturous "It is faine! It is faine!" but he is a private guide. The Bargello custodians belong to the other camp.

The fondness of sculptors for David as a subject is due to the fact that the Florentines, who had spent so much of their time under tyrants and so much of their blood in resisting them, were captivated by the idea of this stripling freeing his compatriots from Goliath and the Philistines. David, as I have said in my remarks on the Piazza della Signoria, stood to them, with Judith, as a champion of liberty. He was alluring also on account of his youth, so attractive to Renaissance sculptors and poets, and the Florentines' admiration was not diminished by the circumstance that his task was a singularly light one, since he never came to close quarters with his antagonist at all and had the Lord of Hosts on his side. A David of mythology, Perseus, another Florentine hero, a stripling with what looked like a formidable enemy, also enjoyed supernatural assistance.

David appealed to the greatest sculptors of all–to Michelangelo, to Donatello, and to Verrocchio; and Michelangelo made two figures, one of which is here and the other at the Accademia, and Donatello two figures, both of which are here, so that, Verrocchio's example being also here, very interesting comparisons are possible.

Personally I put Michelangelo's small David first; it is the one in which, apart from its beauty, you can best believe. His colossal David seems to me one of the most glorious things in the world; but it is not David; not the simple, ruddy shepherd lad of the Bible. This David could obviously defeat anybody. Donatello's more famous David, in the hat, upstairs, is the most charming creature you ever saw, but it had been far better to call him something else. Both he and Verrocchio's David, also upstairs, are young tournament nobles rather than shepherd lads who have slung a stone at a Philistine bully. I see them both–but particularly perhaps Verrocchio's–in the intervals of strife most acceptably holding up a lady's train, or lying at her feet reading one of Boccaccio's stories; neither could ever have watched a flock. Donatello's second David, behind the more famous one, has more reality; but I would put Michelangelo's smaller one first. And what beautiful marble it is–so rich and warm!

One point which both Donatello's and Verrocchio's David emphasizes is the gulf that was fixed between the Biblical and religious conception of the youthful psalmist and that of these sculptors of the Renaissance. One can, indeed, never think of Donatello as a religious artist. Serious, yes; but not religious, or at any rate not religious in the too common sense of the word, in the sense of appertaining to a special reverential mood distinguished from ordinary moods of dailiness. His David, as I have said, is a comely, cultured boy, who belongs to the very flower of chivalry and romance. Verrocchio's is akin to him, but he has less radiant mastery. Donatello's David might be the young lord; Verrocchio's, his page. Here we see the new spirit, the Renaissance, at work, for though religion called it into being and the Church continued to be its patron, it rapidly divided into two halves, and while the painters were bringing all their genius to glorify sacred history, the scholars were endeavouring to humanize it. In this task they had no such allies as the sculptors, and particularly Donatello, who, always thinking independently and vigorously, was their best friend. Donatello's David fought also more powerfully for the modern spirit (had he known it) than ever he could have done in real life with such a large sword in such delicate hands; for by being the first nude statue of a Biblical character, he made simpler the way to all humanists in whatever medium they worked.

Michelangelo was not often tender. Profoundly sad he could be: indeed his own head, in bronze, at the Accademia, might stand for melancholy and bitter world-knowledge; but seldom tender; yet the Madonna and Child in the circular bas-relief in this ground-floor room have something very nigh tenderness, and a greatness that none of the other Italian sculptors, however often they attempted this subject, ever reached. The head of Mary in this relief is, I think, one of the most beautiful things in Florence, none the less so for the charming head-dress which the great austere artist has given her. The Child is older than is usual in such groups, and differs in another way, for tiring of a reading lesson, He has laid His arm upon the book: a pretty touch.

Michelangelo's Bacchus, an early work, is opposite. It is a remarkable proof of his extraordinary range that the same little room should contain the David, the Madonna, the Brutus, and the Bacchus. In David one can believe, as I have said, as the young serious stalwart of the Book of Kings. The Madonna, although perhaps a shade too intellectual–or at any rate more intellectual and commanding than the other great artists have accustomed us to think of her–has a sweet gravity and power and almost domestic tenderness. The Brutus is powerful and modern and realistic; while Bacchus is steeped in the Greek spirit, and the little faun hiding behind him is the very essence of mischief. Add to these the fluid vigour of the unfinished relief of the Martyrdom of S. Andrew, No. 126, and you have five examples of human accomplishment that would be enough without the other Florentine evidences at all–the Medici chapel tombs and the Duomo Pieta.

The inscription under the Brutus says: "While the sculptor was carving the statue of Brutus in marble, he thought of the crime and held his hand"; and the theory is that Michelangelo was at work upon this head at Rome when, in 1537, Lorenzino de' Medici, who claimed to be a modern Brutus, murdered Alessandro de' Medici. But it might easily have been that the sculptor was concerned only with Brutus the friend of Cæsar and revolted at his crime. The circumstance that the head is unfinished matters nothing. Once seen it can never be forgotten.

Although Michelangelo is, as always, the dominator, this room has other possessions to make it a resort of visitors. At the end is a fireplace from the

Casa Borgherini, by Benedetto da Rovezzano, which probably has not an equal, although the pietra serena of which it is made is a horrid hue; and on the walls are fragments of the tomb of S. Giovanni Gualberto at Vallombrosa, designed by the same artist but never finished. Benedetto (1474-1556) has a peculiar interest to the English in having come to England in 1524 at the bidding of Cardinal Wolsey to design a tomb for that proud prelate. On Wolsey's disgrace, Henry VIII decided that the tomb should be continued for his own bones; but the sculptor died first and it was unfinished. Later Charles I cast envious eyes upon it and wished to lie within it; but circumstances deprived him too of the honour. Finally, after having been despoiled of certain bronze additions, the sarcophagus was used for the remains of Nelson, which it now holds, in St. Paul's crypt. The Borgherini fireplace is a miracle of exquisite work, everything having received thought, the delicate traceries on the pillars not less than the frieze. The fireplace is in perfect condition, not one head having been knocked off, but the Gualberto reliefs are badly damaged, yet full of life. The angel under the saint's bier in No. 104 almost moves.

In this room look also at the beautiful blades of barley on the pillars in the corner close to Brutus, and the lovely frieze by an unknown hand above Michelangelo's Martyrdom of S. Andrew, and the carving upon the two niches for statues on either side of the door.

The little room through which one passes to the Michelangelos may well be lingered in. There is a gravely fine floor-tomb of a nun to the left of the door–No. 20–which one would like to see in its proper position instead of upright against the wall; and a stone font in the middle which is very fine. There is also a beautiful tomb by Giusti da Settignano, and the iron gates are worth attention.

From Michelangelo let us ascend the stairs, past the splendid gates, to Donatello; and here a word about that sculptor, for though we meet him again and again in Florence (yet never often enough) it is in the upper room in the Bargello that he is enthroned. Of Donatello there is nothing known but good, and good of the most captivating variety. Not only was he a great creative genius, equally the first modern sculptor and the sanest, but he was himself tall and comely, open-handed, a warm friend, humorous and of vigorous intellect. A hint of the affection in which he was held is obtained from his name Donatello, which is a pet diminutive of Donato–his full style being Donato di Niccolò di Betto Bardi. Born in 1386, four years before Fra Angelico and nearly a century after Giotto, he was the son of a well-to-do woolcomber who was no stranger to the perils of political energy in these times. Of Donatello's youth little is known, but it is almost certain that he helped Ghiberti with his first Baptistery doors, being thirteen when that sculptor began upon them. At sixteen he was himself enrolled as a sculptor. It was soon after this that, as I have said in the first chapter, he accompanied his friend Brunelleschi, who was thirteen years his senior, to Rome; and returning alone he began work in Florence in earnest, both for the cathedral and campanile and for Or San Michele. In 1425 he took into partnership Michelozzo, and became, with him, a protégé of Cosimo de' Medici, with whom both continued on friendly terms for the rest of their lives. In 1433 he was in Rome again, probably not sorry to be there since Cosimo had been banished and had taken Michelozzo with him. On the triumphant return of Cosimo in 1434 Donatello's most prosperous period began; for he was intimate with the most powerful man in Florence, was honoured by him, and was himself at the useful age of forty-four.

Of Donatello as an innovator I have said something above, in considering the Florentine Davids, but he was also the inventor of that low relief in which his school worked, called rilievo stiacciato, of which there are some excellent examples at South Kensington. In Ghiberti's high relief, breaking out often into completely detached figures, he was also a master, as we shall see at S. Lorenzo. But his greatest claim to distinction is his psychological insight allied to perfect mastery of form. His statues were not only the first really great statues since the Greeks, but are still (always leaving Michelangelo on one side as abnormal) the greatest modern examples judged upon a realistic basis. Here in the Bargello, in originals and in casts, he may be adequately appreciated; but to Padua his admirers must certainly go, for the bronze equestrian statue of Gattamelata is there. Donatello was painted by his friend Masaccio at the Carmine, but the fresco has perished. He is to be seen in the Uffizi portico, although that is probably a fancy representation; and again on a tablet in the wall opposite the apse of the Duomo. The only contemporary portrait (and this is very doubtful) is in a picture in the Louvre given to Uccello–a serious, thoughtful, bearded face with steady, observant eyes: one of five heads, the others being Giotto, Manetti, Brunelleschi, and Uccello himself.

Donatello, who never married, but lived for much of his life with his mother and sister, died at a great age, cared for both by Cosimo de' Medici and his son and successor Piero. He was buried with Cosimo in S. Lorenzo. Vasari tells us that he was free, affectionate, and courteous, but of a high spirit and capable of sudden anger, as when he destroyed with a blow a head he had made for a mean patron who objected to its very reasonable price. "He thought," says Vasari, "nothing of money, keeping it in a basket suspended from the ceiling, so that all his workmen and friends took what they wanted without saying anything." He was as careless of dress as great artists have ever been, and of a handsome robe which Cosimo gave him he complained that it spoiled his work. When he was dying his relations affected great concern in the hope of inheriting a farm at Prato, but he told them that he had left it to the peasant who had always toiled there, and he would not alter his will.

The Donatello collection in the Bargello has been made representative by the addition of casts. The originals number ten: there is also a cast of the equestrian statue of Gattemalata at Padua, which is, I suppose, next to Verrocchio's Bartolommeo Colleoni at Venice, the finest equestrian statue that exists; heads from various collections, including M. Dreyfus' in Paris, although Dr. Bode now gives that charming example to Donatello's pupil Desiderio; and various other masterpieces elsewhere. But it is the originals that chiefly interest us, and first of these in bronze is the David, of which I have already spoken, and first of these in marble the S. George. This George is just such a resolute, clean, warlike idealist as one dreams him. He would kill a dragon, it is true; but he would eat and sleep after it and tell the story modestly and not without humour. By a happy chance the marble upon which Donatello worked had light veins running through it just where the head is, with the result that the face seems to possess a radiance of its own. This statue was made for Or San Michele, where it used to stand until 1891, when the present bronze replica that takes its place was made. The spirited marble frieze underneath it at Or San Michele is the original and has been there for centuries. It was this S. George whom Ruskin took as the head and inspiration of his Saint George's Guild.

The David is interesting not only in itself but as being the first isolated statue of modern times. It was made for Cosimo de' Medici, to stand in the courtyard of the Medici palace (now the Riccardi), and until that time, since antiquity, no one had made a statue to stand on a pedestal and be observable from all points. Hitherto modern sculptors had either made reliefs or statues for niches. It was also the first nude statue of modern times; and once again one has the satisfaction of recognizing that the first was the best. At any rate, no later sculptor has made anything more charming than this figure, or more masterly within its limits.

After the S. George and the bronze David, the two most memorable things are the adorable bronze Amorino in its quaint little trousers–or perhaps not Amorino at all, since it is trampling on a snake, which such little sprites did not do–and the coloured terra-cotta bust called Niccolò da Uzzano, so like life as to be after a while disconcerting. The sensitiveness of the mouth can never have been excelled. The other originals include the gaunt John the Baptist with its curious little moustache, so far removed from the Amorino and so admirable a proof of the sculptor's vigilant thoughtfulness in all he did; the relief of the infant John, one of the most animated of the heads (the Baptist at all periods of his life being a favourite with this sculptor); three bronze heads, of which those of the Young Gentleman and the Roman

Emperor remain most clearly in my mind. But the authorship of the Roman Emperor is very doubtful. And lastly the glorious Marzocco–the lion from the front of the Palazzo Vecchio, firmly holding the Florentine escutcheon against the world. Florence has other Donatellos–the Judith in the Loggia de' Lanzi, the figures on Giotto's campanile, the Annunciation in S. Croce, and above all the cantoria in the Museum of the Cathedral; but this room holds most of his strong sweet genius. Here (for there are seldom more than two or three persons in it) you can be on terms with him.

After the Donatellos we should see the other Renaissance sculpture. But first the Carrand collection of ivories, pictures, jewels, carvings, vestments, plaquettes, and objets d'art, bequeathed to Florence in 1888. Everything here is good and worth examination. Among the outstanding things is a plaquette, No. 393, a Satyr and a Bacchante, attributed to Donatello, under the title "Allegory of Spring," which is the work of a master and a very riot of mythological imagery. The neighbouring plaquettes, many of them of the school of Donatello, are all beautiful.

We now find the sixth salon, to see Verrocchio's David, of which I have already spoken. This wholly charming boy, a little nearer life perhaps than Donatello's, although not quite so radiantly distinguished, illustrates the association of Verrocchio and Leonardo as clearly as any of the paintings do; for the head is sheer Leonardo. At the Palazzo Vecchio we saw Verrocchio's boy with the dolphin–that happy bronze lyric–and outside Or San Michele his Christ and S. Thomas, in Donatello and Michelozzo's niche, with the flying cherubim beneath. But as with Donatello, so with Verrocchio, one must visit the Bargello to see him, in Florence, most intimately. For here are not only his David, which once known can never be forgotten and is as full of the Renaissance spirit as anything ever fashioned, whether in bronze, marble, or paint, but–upstairs–certain other wonderfully beautiful things to which we shall come, and, that being so, I would like here to say a little about their author.

Verrocchio is a nickname, signifying the true eye. Andrea's real name was de' Cioni; he is known to fame as Andrea of the true eye, and since he had acquired this style at a time when every eye was true enough, his must have been true indeed. It is probable that he was a pupil of Donatello, who in 1435, when Andrea was born, was forty-nine, and in time he was to become the master of Leonardo: thus are the great artists related. The history of Florentine art is practically the history of a family; one artist leads to the other–the genealogy of genius. The story goes that it was the excellence of the angel contributed by Leonardo to his master's picture of the Baptism of Christ (at the Accademia) which decided Verrocchio to paint no more, just as Ghiberti's superiority in the relief of Abraham and Isaac drove Brunelleschi from sculpture. If this be so, it accounts for the extraordinarily small number of pictures by him. Like many artists of his day Verrocchio was also a goldsmith, but he was versatile above most, even when versatility was a habit, and excelled also as a musician. Both Piero de' Medici and Lorenzo employed him to design their tournament costumes; and it was for Lorenzo that he made this charming David and the boy and the dolphin. His greatest work of all is the bronze equestrian statue of Bartolommeo Colleoni in Venice, the finest thing of its kind in the world, and so glorious and exciting indeed that every city should have a cast of it in a conspicuous position just for the good of the people. It was while at work upon this that Verrocchio died, at the age of fifty-three. His body was brought from Venice by his pupil Lorenzo di Credi, who adored him, and was buried in S. Ambrogio in Florence. Lorenzo di Credi painted his portrait, which is now in the Uffizi–a plump, undistinguished-looking little man.

In the David room are also the extremely interesting rival bronze reliefs of Abraham sacrificing Isaac, which were made by Ghiberti and Brunelleschi as trials of skill to see which would win the commission to design the new gates of the Baptistery, as I have told earlier in this book. Six competitors entered for the contest; but Ghiberti's and Brunelleschi's efforts were alone considered seriously. A comparison of these two reliefs proves that Ghiberti, at any rate, had a finer sense of grouping. He filled the space at his disposal more easily and his hand was more fluent; but there is a very engaging vivacity in the other work, the realistic details of which are so arresting as to make one regret that Brunelleschi had for sculpture so little time. In S. Maria Novella is that crucifix in wood which he carved for his friend Donatello, but his only other sculptured work in Florence is the door of his beautiful Pazzi chapel in the cloisters of S. Croce. Of Ghiberti's Baptistery gates I have said more elsewhere. Enough here to add that the episode of Abraham and Isaac does not occur in them.

This little room also has a Cassa Reliquiaria by Ghiberti, below a fine relief by Bertoldo, Michelangelo's master in sculpture, representing a battle between the Romans and the Barbarians; cases of exquisite bronzes; the head, in bronze (No. 25), of an old placid, shrewd woman, executed from a death-mask, which the photographers call Contessina de' Bardi, wife of Cosimo de' Medici, by Donatello, but which cannot be so, since the sculptor died first; heads of Apollo and two babies, over the Ghiberti and Brunelleschi competition reliefs; a crucifixion by Bertoldo; a row of babies representing the triumph of Bacchus; and below these a case of medals and plaquettes, every one a masterpiece.

The next room, Sala VII, is apportioned chiefly between Cellini and Gian or Giovanni da Bologna, the two sculptors who dominate the Loggia de' Lanzi. Here we may see models for Cellini's Perseus in bronze and wax and also for the relief of the rescue of Andromeda, under the statue; his Cosimo I, with the wart (omitted by Bandinelli in the head downstairs, which pairs with Michelangelo's Brutus); and various smaller works. But personally I find that Cellini will not do in such near proximity to Donatello, Verrocchio, and their gentle followers. He was, of course, far later. He was not born (in 1500) until Donatello had been dead thirty-four years, Mino da Fiesole sixteen years, Desiderio da Settignano thirty-six years, and Verrocchio twelve years. He thus did not begin to work until the finer impulses of the Renaissance were exhausted. Giovanni da Bologna, although he, it is true, was even later (1524-1608), I find more sympathetic; while Landor boldly proclaimed him superior to Michelangelo. His "Mercury," in the middle of the room, which one sees counterfeited in all the statuary shops of Florence, is truly very nearly light as air. If ever bronze floated, this figure does. His cherubs and dolphins are very skilful and merry; his turkey and eagle and other animals indicate that he had humility. John of Bologna is best known at Florence by his Rape of the Sabines and Hercules and Nessus in the Loggia de' Lanzi; but the Boboli gardens have a fine group of Oceanus and river gods by him in the midst of a lake. Before leaving this room look at the relief of Christ in glory (No. 35), to the left of the door, by Jacopo Sansovino, a rival of Michelangelo, which is most admirable, and at the case of bronze animals by Pietro Tacca, John of Bologna's pupil, who made the famous boar (a copy of an ancient marble) at the Mercato Nuovo and the reliefs for the pediment of the statue of Cosimo I (by his master) in the Piazza della Signoria. But I believe that the most beautiful thing in this room is the bronze figure for the tomb of Mariano Sozzino by Lorenzo di Pietro.

Before we look at the della Robbias, which are in the two large rooms upstairs, let us finish with the marble and terra-cotta statuary in the two smaller rooms to the left as one passes through the first della Robbia room. In the first of them, corresponding to the room with Verrocchio's David downstairs, we find Verrocchio again, with a bust of Piero di Lorenzo de' Medici (whom Botticelli painted in the Uffizi holding a medal in his hand) and a most exquisite Madonna and Child in terra-cotta from S. Maria Nuova. (This is on a hinge, for better light, but the official skies will fall if you touch it.) Here also is the bust of a young warrior by Antonio Pollaiuolo (1429-1498) who was Verrocchio's closest rival and one of Ghiberti's assistants for the second Baptistery doors. His greatest work is at Rome, but this bust is indescribably charming, and the softness of the boy's contours is almost of life. It is sometimes called Giuliano de' Medici. Other beautiful objects in the room are the terra-cotta Madonna and Child by Andrea Sansovino (1460-1529), Pollaiuolo's pupil, which is as radiant although not so domestically lovely as Verrocchio's; the bust by Benedetto da Maiano (1442-1497) of Pietro Mellini, that shrewd and wrinkled patron of the Church who presented to S. Croce the famous pulpit by this sculptor; an ancient lady, by the door, in coloured terra-cotta, who is thought to represent Monna Tessa, the nurse of Dante's Beatrice; and certain other works by that delightful and prolific person Ignoto Fiorentino, who here, and in the next room, which we now enter, is at his best.

This next priceless room is chiefly memorable for Verrocchio and Mino da Fiesole. We come to Verrocchio at once, on the left, where his relief of the death of Francesca Pitti Tornabuoni (on a tiny bed only half as long as herself) may be seen. This poor lady, who died in childbirth, was the wife of Giovanni Tornabuoni, and he it was who employed Ghirlandaio to make the frescoes in the choir of S. Maria Novella. (I ought, however, to state that Miss Cruttwell, in her monograph on Verrocchio, questions both the subject and the artist.) Close by we have two more works by Verrocchio–No. 180, a marble relief of the Madonna and Child, the Madonna's dress fastened by the prettiest of brooches, and She herself possessing a dainty sad head and the long fingers that Verrocchio so favoured, which we find again in the famous "Gentildonna" (No. 181) next it–that Florentine lady with flowers in her bosom, whose contours are so exquisite and who has such pretty shoulders.

Near by is the little eager S. John the Baptist as a boy by Antonio Rossellino (1427-1478), and on the next wall the same sculptor's circular relief of the Madonna adoring, in a border of cherubs. In the middle is the masterpiece of Jacopo Sansovino (1486-1570): a Bacchus, so strangely like a genuine antique, full of Greek lightness and grace. And then we come back to the wall in which the door is, and find more works from the delicate hand of Mino da Fiesole, whom we in London are fortunate in being able to study as near home as at the Victoria and Albert Museum. Of Mino I have said more both at the Badia and at Fiesole. But here I might remark again that he was born in 1431 and died in 1484, and was the favourite pupil of Desiderio da Settignano, who was in his turn the favourite pupil of Donatello.

In the little church of S. Ambrogio we have seen a tablet to the memory of Mino, who lies there, not far from the grave of Verrocchio, whom he most nearly approached in feeling, although their ideal type of woman differed in everything save the slenderness of the fingers. The Bargello has both busts and reliefs by him, all distinguished and sensitive and marked by Mino's profound refinement. The Madonna and Child in No. 232 are peculiarly beautiful and notable both for high relief and shallow relief, and the Child in No. 193 is even more charming. For delicacy and vivacity in marble portraiture it would be impossible to surpass the head of Rinaldo della Luna; and the two Medicis are wonderfully real. Everything in Mino's work is thoughtful and exquisite, while the unusual type of face which so attracted him gives him freshness too.

This room and that next it illustrate the wealth of fine sculptors which Florence had in the fifteenth century, for the works by the unknown hands are in some cases hardly less beautiful and masterly than those by the known. Look, for example, at the fleur-de-lis over the door; at the Madonna and Child next it, on the right; at the girl's head next to that; at the baby girl at the other end of the room; and at the older boy and his pendant. But one does not need to come here to form an idea of the wealth of good sculpture. The streets alone are full of it. Every palace has beautiful stone-work and an escutcheon which often only a master could execute–as Donatello devised that for the Palazzo Pazzi in the Borgo degli Albizzi. On the great staircase of the Bargello, for example, are numbers of coats of arms that could not be more beautifully designed and incised.

In the room leading from that which is memorable for Pollaiuolo's youth in armour is a collection of medals by all the best medallists, beginning, in the first case, with Pisanello. Here are his Sigismondo Malatesta, the tyrant of Rimini, and Isotta his wife; here also is a portrait of Leon Battista Alberti, who designed and worked on the cathedral of Rimini as well as upon S. Maria Novella in Florence. On the other side of this case is the medal commemorating the Pazzi conspiracy. In other cases are pretty Italian ladies, such as Julia Astalla, Lucrezia Tornabuoni, with her hair in curls just as in Ghirlandaio's frescoes, Costanza Rucellai, Leonora Altoviti, Maria Poliziano, and Maria de' Mucini.

And so we come to the della Robbias, without whose joyous, radiant art Florence would be only half as beautiful as she is. Of these exquisite artists Luca, the uncle, born in 1400, was by far the greatest. Andrea, his nephew, born in 1435, came next, and then Giovanni. Luca seems to have been a serious, quiet man who would probably have made sculpture not much below his friend Donatello's had not he chanced on the discovery of a means of colouring and glazing terra-cotta. Examples of this craft are seen all over Florence both within doors and out, as the pages of this book indicate, but at the Bargello is the greatest number of small pieces gathered together. I do not say there is anything here more notable than the Annunciation attributed to Andrea at the Spedale degli Innocenti, while of course, for most people, his putti on the façade of that building are the della Robbia symbol; nor is there anything finer than Luca's work at Impruneta; but as a collection of sweetness and gentle domestic beauty these Bargello reliefs are unequalled, both in character and in volume. Here you see what one might call Roman Catholic art–that is, the art which at once gives pleasure to simple souls and symbolizes benevolence and safety–carried out to its highest power. Tenderness, happiness, and purity are equally suggested by every relief here. Had Luca and Andrea been entrusted with the creation of the world it would be a paradise. And, as it is, it seems to me impossible but that they left the world sweeter than they found it. Such examples of affection and solicitude as they were continually bringing to the popular vision must have engendered kindness.

I have noted as especially beautiful in the first room Nos. 4, 6, 12, 23, by Andrea; and 10 and 21, by Luca. These, by the way, are the Bargello ascriptions, but the experts do not always agree. Herr Bode, for example, who has studied the della Robbias with passionate thoroughness, gives the famous head of the boy, which is in reproduction one of the best-known works of plastic art, to Luca; but the Bargello director says Andrea. In Herr Bode's fascinating monograph, "Florentine Sculptors of the Renaissance," he goes very carefully into the differences between the uncle and the nephew, master and pupil. In all the groups, for example, he says that Luca places the Child on the Madonna's left arm, Andrea on the right. In the second room I have marked particularly Nos. 21, 28, and 31, by Luca, 28 being a deeper relief than usual, and the Madonna not adoring but holding and delighting in one of the most adorable of Babies. Observe in the reproduction of this relief in this volume– how the Mother's fingers sink into the child's flesh. Luca was the first sculptor to notice that. No. 31 is the lovely Madonna of the Rose Bower. But nothing gives me more pleasure than the boy's head of which I have just spoken, attributed to Andrea and also reproduced here. The "Giovane Donna" which pairs with it has extraordinary charm and delicacy too. I have marked also, by Andrea, Nos. 71 and 76. Giovanni della Robbia's best is perhaps No. 15, in the other room.

One curious thing that one notes about della Robbia pottery is its inability to travel. It was made for the church and it should remain there. Even in the Bargello, where there is an ancient environment, it loses half its charm; while in an English museum it becomes hard and cold. But in a church to which the poor carry their troubles, with a dim light and a little incense, it is perfect, far beyond painting in its tenderness and symbolic value. I speak of course of the Madonnas and altar-pieces. When the della Robbias worked for the open air–as in the façade of the Children's Hospital, or at the Certosa, or in the Loggia di San Paolo, opposite S. Maria Novella, where one may see the beautiful meeting of S. Francis and S. Dominic, by Andrea–they seem, in Italy, to have fitness enough; but it would not do to transplant any of these reliefs to an English façade. There was once, I might add, in Florence a Via della Robbia, but it is now the Via Nazionale. I suppose this injustice to the great potters came about in the eighteen-sixties, when popular political enthusiasm led to every kind of similar re-naming.

In the room leading out of the second della Robbia room is a collection of vestments and brocades bequeathed by Baron Giulio Franchetti, where you may see, dating from as far back as the sixth century, designs that for beauty and splendour and durability put to shame most of the stuffs now woven; but the top floor of the Museo Archeologico in the Via della Colonna is the chief home in Florence of such treasures.

There are other beautiful things in the Bargello of which I have said nothing–a gallery of mediaeval bells most exquisitely designed, from famous steeples; cases of carved ivory; and many of such treasures as one sees at the Cluny in Paris. But it is for its courtyard and for the Renaissance sculpture that one goes to the Bargello, and returns again and again to the Bargello, and it is for these that one remembers it.

On returning to London the first duty of every one who has drunk deep of delight in the Bargello is to visit that too much neglected treasure-house of our own, the Victoria and Albert Museum at South Kensington. There may be nothing at South Kensington as fine as the Bargello's finest, but it is a priceless collection and is superior to the Bargello in one respect at any rate, for it has a relief attributed to Leonardo. Here also is an adorable Madonna and laughing Child, beyond anything in Florence for sheer gaiety if not mischief, which the South Kensington authorities call a Rossellino but Herr Bode a Desiderio da Settignano. The room is rich too in Donatello and in Verrocchio, and altogether it makes a perfect footnote to the Bargello. It also has within call learned gentlemen who can give intimate information about the exhibits, which the Bargello badly lacks. The Louvre and the Kaiser Friedrich Museum in Berlin–but particularly the Kaiser Friedrich since Herr Bode, who has such a passion for this period, became its director–have priceless treasures, and in Paris I have had the privilege of seeing the little but exquisite collection formed by M. Gustave Dreyfus, dominated by that mirthful Italian child which the Bargello authorities consider to be by Donatello, but Herr Bode gives to Desiderio. At the Louvre, in galleries on the ground floor gained through the Egyptian sculpture section and opened very capriciously, may be seen the finest of the prisoners from Michelangelo's tomb for Pope Julius; Donatello's youthful Baptist; a Madonna and Children by Agostino di Duccio, whom we saw at the Museum of the Cathedral; an early coloured terra-cotta by Luca della Robbia, and No. 316, a terra-cotta Madonna and Child without ascription, which looks very like Rossellino.

In addition to originals there are at South Kensington casts of many of the Bargello's most valuable possessions, such as Donatello's and Verrocchio's Davids, Donatello's Baptist and many heads, Mino da Fiesole's best Madonna, Pollaiuolo's Young Warrior, and so forth; so that to loiter there is most attractively to recapture something of the Florentine feeling.

CHAPTER XV

. Croce

S
An historic piazza–Marble façades–Florence's Westminster Abbey–Galileo's ancestor and Ruskin–Benedetto's pulpit–Michelangelo's tomb–A fond lady–Donatello's Annunciation–Giotto's frescoes–S. Francis–Donatello magnanimous–The gifted Alberti–Desiderio's great tomb–The sacristy–The Medici chapel–The Pazzi chapel–Old Jacopo desecrated–A Restoration.

The piazza S. Croce now belongs to children. The church is at one end, bizarre buildings are on either side, the Dante statue is in the middle, and harsh gravel covers the ground. Everywhere are children, all dirty, and all rather squalid and mostly bow-legged, showing that they were of the wrong age to take their first steps on Holy Saturday at noon. The long brown building on the right, as we face S. Croce, is a seventeenth-century palazzo. For the rest, the architecture is chiefly notable for green shutters.

The frigid and florid Dante memorial, which was unveiled in 1865 on the six hundredth anniversary of the poet's birthday, looks gloomily upon what once was a scene of splendour and animation, for in 1469 Piero de' Medici devised here a tournament in honour of the betrothal of Lorenzo to Clarice

Orsini. The Queen of the tournament was Lucrezia Donati, and she awarded the first prize to Lorenzo. The tournament cost 10,000 gold florins and was very splendid, Verrocchio and other artists being called in to design costumes, and it is thought that Pollaiuolo's terra-cotta of the Young Warrior in the Bargello represents the comely Giuliano de' Medici as he appeared in his armour in the lists. The piazza was the scene also of that famous tournament given by Lorenzo de' Medici for Giuliano in 1474, of which the beautiful Simonetta was the Queen of Beauty, and to which, as I have said elsewhere, we owe Botticelli's two most famous pictures. Difficult to reconstruct in the Piazza any of those glories to-day.

The new façade of S. Croce, endowed not long since by an Englishman, has been much abused, but it is not so bad. As the front of so beautiful and wonderful a church it may be inadequate, but as a structure of black and white marble it will do. To my mind nothing satisfactory can now be done in this medium, which, unless it is centuries old, is always harsh and cuts the sky like a knife, instead of resting against it as architecture should. But when it is old, as at S. Miniato, it is right.

S. Croce is the Westminster Abbey of Florence. Michelangelo lies here, Machiavelli lies here, Galileo lies here; and here Giotto painted, Donatello carved, and Brunelleschi planned. Although outside the church is disappointing, within it is the most beautiful in Florence. It has the boldest arches, the best light at all seasons, the most attractive floor–of gentle red–and an apse almost wholly made of coloured glass. Not a little of its charm comes from the delicate passage-way that runs the whole course of the church high up on the yellow walls. It also has the finest circular window in Florence, over the main entrance, a "Deposition" by Ghiberti.

The lightness was indeed once so intense that no fewer than twenty-two windows had to be closed. The circular window over the altar upon which a new roof seems to be intruding is in reality the interloper: the roof is the original one, and the window was cut later, in defiance of good architecture, by Vasari, who, since he was a pupil of Michelangelo, should have known better. To him was entrusted the restoration of the church in the middle of the sixteenth century.

The original architect of the modern S. Croce was the same Arnolfo di Cambio, or Lapo, who began the Duomo. He had some right to be chosen since his father, Jacopo, or Lapo, a German, was the builder of the most famous of all the Franciscan churches–that at Assisi, which was begun while S. Francis was still living. And Giotto, who painted in that church his most famous frescoes, depicting scenes in the life of S. Francis, succeeded Arnolfo here, as at the Duomo, with equal fitness. Arnolfo began S. Croce in 1294, the year that the building of the Duomo was decided upon, as a reply to the new Dominican Church of S. Maria Novella, and to his German origin is probably due the Northern impression which the interiors both of S. Croce and the Duomo convey.

The first thing to examine in S. Croce is the floor-tomb, close to the centre door, upon which Ruskin wrote one of his most characteristic passages. The tomb is of an ancestor of Galileo (who lies close by, but beneath a florid monument), and it represents a mediaeval scholarly figure with folded hands. Ruskin writes: "That worn face is still a perfect portrait of the old man, though like one struck out at a venture, with a few rough touches of a master's chisel. And that falling drapery of his cap is, in its few lines, faultless, and subtle beyond description. And now, here is a simple but most useful test of your capacity for understanding Florentine sculpture or painting. If you can see that the lines of that cap are both right, and lovely; that the choice of the folds is exquisite in its ornamental relations of line; and that the softness and ease of them is complete,–though only sketched with a few dark touches,–then you can understand Giotto's drawing, and Botticelli's; Donatello's carving and Luca's. But if you see nothing in this sculpture, you will see nothing in theirs, of theirs. Where they choose to imitate flesh, or silk, or to play any vulgar modern trick with marble–(and they often do)–whatever, in a word, is French, or American, or Cockney, in their work, you can see; but what is Florentine, and for ever great–unless you can see also the beauty of this old man in his citizen's cap,–you will see never."

The passage is in "Mornings in Florence," which begins with S. Croce and should be read by every one visiting the city. And here let me advise another companion for this church: a little dark enthusiast, in a black skull cap, named Alfred Branconi, who is usually to be found just inside the doors, but may be secured as a guide by a postcard to the church. Signor Branconi knows S. Croce and he loves it, and he has the further qualifications of knowing all Florence too and speaking excellent English, which he taught himself.

The S. Croce pulpit, which is by Benedetto da Maiano, is a satisfying thing, accomplished both in proportions and workmanship, with panels illustrating scenes in the life of S. Francis. These are all most gently and persuasively done, influenced, of course, by the Baptistery doors, but individual too, and full of a kindred sweetness and liveliness. The scenes are the "Confirmation of the Franciscan Order" (the best, I think); the "Burning of the Books"; the "Stigmata," which we shall see again in the church, in fresco, for here we are all dedicated to the saint of Assisi, not yet having come upon the stern S. Dominic, the ruler at S. Marco and S. Maria Novella; the "Death of S. Francis," very real and touching, which we shall also see again; and the execution of certain Franciscans. Benedetto, who was also an architect and made the plan of the Strozzi palace, was so unwilling that anything should mar the scheme of his pulpit, that after strengthening this pillar with the greatest care and thoroughness, he hollowed it and placed the stairs inside.

The first tomb on the right, close to this pulpit, is Michelangelo's, a mass of allegory, designed by his friend Vasari, the author of the "Lives of the Artists," the reading of which is perhaps the best preparation for the understanding of Florence. "If life pleases us," Michelangelo once said, "we ought not to be grieved by death, which comes from the same Giver." Michelangelo had intended the Pietà, now in the Duomo, to stand above his grave; but Vasari, who had a little of the Pepys in his nature, thought to do him greater honour by this ornateness. The artist was laid to his rest in 1564, but not before his body was exhumed, by his nephew, at Rome, where the great man had died, and a series of elaborate ceremonies had been performed, which Vasari, who is here trustworthy enough, describes minutely. All the artists in Florence vied in celebrating the dead master in memorial paintings for his catafalque and its surroundings, which have now perished; but probably the loss is not great, except as an example of homage, for that was a bad period. How bad it was may be a little gauged by Vasari's tributory tomb and his window over the high altar.

Opposite Michelangelo's tomb, on the pillar, is the pretty but rather Victorian "Madonna del Latte," surrounded by angels, by Bernardo Rossellino (1409-1464), brother of the author of the great tomb at S. Miniato. This pretty relief was commissioned as a family memorial by that Francesco Nori, the close friend of Lorenzo de' Medici, who was killed in the Duomo during the Pazzi conspiracy in his effort to save Lorenzo from the assassins.

The tomb of Alfieri, the dramatist, to which we now come, was erected at the cost of his mistress, the Countess of Albany, who herself sat to Canova for the figure of bereaved Italy. This curious and unfortunate woman became, at the age of nineteen, the wife of the Young Pretender, twenty-seven years after the '45, and led a miserable existence with him (due chiefly to his depravity, but a little, she always held, to the circumstance that they chose Good Friday for their wedding day) until Alfieri fell in love with her and offered his protection. Together she and the poet remained, apparently contented with each other and received by society, even by the English Royal family, until Alfieri died, in 1803, when after exclaiming that she had lost all–"consolations, support, society, all, all!"–and establishing this handsome memorial, she selected the French artist Fabre to fill the aching void in her fifty-years-old heart; and Fabre not only filled it until her death in 1824, but became the heir of all that had been bequeathed to her by both the Stuart and Alfieri. Such was the Countess of Albany, to whom human affection was so necessary. She herself is buried close by, in the chapel of the Castellani.

Mrs. Piozzi, in her "Glimpses of Italian Society," mentions seeing in Florence in 1785 the unhappy Pretender. Though old and sickly, he went much into society, sported the English arms and livery, and wore the garter.

Other tombs in the right aisle are those of Machiavelli, the statesman and author of "The Prince," and Rossini, the composer of "William Tell," who died in Paris in 1868, but was brought here for burial. These tombs are modern and of no artistic value, but there is near them a fine fifteenth-century example in the monument by Bernardo Rossellino to another statesman and author, Leonardo Bruni, known as Aretino, who wrote the lives of Dante and Petrarch and a Latin history of Florence, a copy of which was placed on his heart at his funeral. This tomb is considered to be Rossellino's masterpiece; but there is one opposite by another hand which dwarfs it.

There is also a work of sculpture near it, in the same wall, which draws away the eyes–Donatello's "Annunciation". The experts now think this to belong to the sculptor's middle period, but Vasari thought it earlier, and makes it the work which had most influence in establishing his reputation; while according to the archives it was placed in the church before Donatello was living. Vasari ought to be better informed upon this point than usual, since it was he who was employed in the sixteenth century to renovate S. Croce, at which time the chapel for whose altar the relief was made–that of the Cavalcanti family–was removed. The relief now stands unrelated to anything. Every detail of it should be examined; but Alfred Branconi will see to that. The stone is the grey pietra serena of Fiesole, and Donatello has plentifully, but not too plentifully, lightened it with gold, which is exactly what all artists who used this medium for sculpture should have done. By a pleasant tactful touch the designer of the modern Donatello monument in S. Lorenzo has followed the master's lead.

Almost everything of Donatello's that one sees is in turn the best; but standing before this lovely work one is more than commonly conscious of being in the presence of a wonderful creator. The Virgin is wholly unlike any other woman, and She is surprising and modern even for Donatello with his vast range. The charming terra-cotta boys above are almost without doubt from the same hand, but they cannot have been made for this monument.

To the della Robbias we come in the Castellani chapel in the right transept, which has two full-length statues by either Luca or Andrea, in the gentle glazed medium, of S. Francis and S. Bernard, quite different from anything we have seen or shall see, because isolated. The other full-size figures by these masters–such as those at Impruneta–are placed against the wall. The S. Bernard, on the left as one enters the chapel, is far the finer. It surely must be one of the most beautiful male draped figures in the world.

The next chapel, at the end of the transept, was once enriched by Giotto frescoes, but they no longer exist. There are, however, an interesting but restored series of scenes in the life of the Virgin by Taddeo Gaddi, Giotto's godson; a Madonna ascending to heaven, by Mainardi, who was Ghirlandaio's pupil, and so satisfactory a one that he was rewarded by the hand of his master's sister; and a pretty piece of Gothic sculpture with the Christ Child upon it. Hereabouts, I may remark, we have continually to be walking over floor-tombs, now ruined beyond hope, their ruin being perhaps the cause of a protecting rail being placed round the others; although a floor-tomb should have, I think, a little wearing from the feet of worshippers, just to soften the lines. Those at the Certosa are, for example, far too sharp and clean.

Let us complete the round of the church before we examine the sacristy, and go now to the two chapels, where Giotto may be found at his best, although restored too, on this side of the high altar. The Peruzzi chapel has scenes from the lives of the two S. Johns, the Baptist, and the Evangelist: all rather too thoroughly re-painted, although following Giotto's groundwork closely enough to retain much of their interest and value. And here once again one should consult the "Mornings in Florence," where the wilful discerning enthusiast is, like his revered subject, also at his best. Giotto's thoughtfulness could not be better illustrated than in S. Croce. One sees him, as ever, thinking of everything: not a very remarkable attribute of the fresco painter since then, but very remarkable then, when any kind of facile saintliness sufficed.

Signor Bianchi, who found these paintings under the whitewash in 1853, and restored them, overdid his part, there is no doubt; but as I have said, their interest is unharmed, and it is that which one so delights in. Look, for instance, at the attitude of Drusiana, suddenly twitched by S. John back again into this vale of tears, while her bier is on its way to the cemetery outside the pretty city. "Am I really to live again?" she so plainly says to the inexorable miracle-worker. The dancing of Herodias' daughter, which offered Giotto less scope, is original too–original not because it came so early, but because Giotto's mind was original and innovating and creative. The musician is charming. The last scene of all is a delightful blend of religious fervour and reality: the miraculous ascent from the tomb, through an elegant Florentine loggia, to everlasting glory, in a blaze of gold, and Christ and an apostle leaning out of heaven with outstretched hands to pull the saint in, as into a boat. Such a Christ as that could not but be believed in.

In the next chapel, the Bardi, we find Giotto at work on a life of S. Francis, and here again Ruskin is essential. It was a task which, since this church was the great effort of the Florentine Franciscans, would put an artist upon his mettle, and Giotto set the chosen incidents before the observers with the discretion and skill of the great biographer that he was, and not only that, but the great Assisi decorator that he was. No choice could have been better at any time in the history of art. Giotto chose the following scenes, one or two of which coincide with those on Benedetto da Maiano's pulpit, which came of course many years later: the "Confirmation of the Rules of the Franciscans," "S. Francis before the Sultan and the Magi," "S. Francis Sick and Appearing to the Bishop of Assisi," "S. Francis Fleeing from His Father's House and His Reception by the Bishop of Assisi," and the "Death of S. Francis". Giotto's Assisi frescoes, which preceded these, anticipate them; but in some cases these are considered to be better, although in others not so good. It is generally agreed that the death scene is the best. Note the characteristic touch by which Giotto makes one of the monks at the head of the bed look up at the precise moment when the saint dies, seeing him being received into heaven. According to Vasari, one of the two monks (on the extreme left, as I suppose) is Giotto's portrait of the architect of the church, Amolfo. The altar picture, consisting of many more scenes in the life of S. Francis, is often attributed to Cimabue, Giotto's master, but probably is by another hand. In one of these scenes the saint is found preaching to what must be the most attentive birds on record. The figures on the ceiling represent Poverty, Chastity, and Obedience, which all Franciscans are pledged to observe. The glass is coeval with the building, which has been described as the most perfect Gothic chapel in existence.

The founder of this chapel was Ridolfo de' Bardi, whose family early in the fourteenth century bade fair to become as powerful as the Medici, and by the same means, their business being banking and money-lending, in association with the founders of the adjoining chapel, the Peruzzi. Ridolfo's father died in 1310, and his son, who had become a Franciscan, in 1327; and the chapel was built, and Giotto probably painted the frescoes, soon after the father's death. Both the Bardi and Peruzzi were brought low by our King Edward III, who borrowed from them money with which to fight the French, at Crecy and Poitiers, and omitted to repay it.

The chapels in the left transept are less interesting, except perhaps to students of painting in its early days. In the chapel at the end we find Donatello's wooden crucifix which led to that friendly rivalry on the part of Brunelleschi, the story of which is one of the best in all Vasari. Donatello, having finished this wooden crucifix, and being unusually satisfied with it, asked Brunelleschi's opinion, confidently expecting praise. But Brunelleschi, who was sufficiently close a friend to say what he thought, replied that the type was too rough and common: it was not Christ but a peasant. Christ, of course, was a peasant; but by peasant Brunelleschi meant a stupid, dull man. Donatello, chagrined, had recourse to what has always been a popular retort to critics, and challenged him to make a better. Brunelleschi took it very quietly: he said nothing in reply, but secretly for many months, in the intervals of his architecture, worked at his own version, and then one day, when it was finished, invited Donatello to dinner, stopping at the Mercato Vecchio to get some eggs and other things. These he gave Donatello to carry, and sent him on before him to the studio, where the crucifix was standing unveiled. When Brunelleschi arrived he found the eggs scattered and broken on the floor and Donatello before his carving in an ecstasy of admiration. "But what are we going to have for dinner?" the host inquired. "Dinner!" said Donatello; "I've had all the dinner I require. To thee it is given to carve Christs: to me only peasants." No one should forget this pretty story, either here or at S. Maria Novella, where Brunelleschi's crucifix now is.

The flexible Siena iron grille of this end chapel dates from 1335. Note its ivy border.

On entering the left aisle we find the tombs of Cherubini, the composer, Raphael Morghen, the engraver, and that curious example of the Florentine universalist, whose figure we saw under the Uffizi, Leon Battista Alberti (1405-1472), architect, painter, author, mathematician, scholar, conversationalist, aristocrat, and friend of princes. His chief work in Florence is the Rucellai palace and the façade of S. Maria Novella, but he was greater as an influence than creator, and his manuals on architecture, painting, and the study of perspective helped to bring the arts to perfection. It is at Rimini that he was perhaps most wonderful. Lorenzo de' Medici greatly valued his society, and he was a leader in the Platonic Academy. But the most human achievement to his credit is his powerful plea for using the vernacular in literature, rather than concealing one's best thoughts, as was fashionable before his protest, in Latin. So much for Alberti's intellectual side. Physically he was remarkable too, and one of his accomplishments was to jump over a man standing upright, while he was also able to throw a coin on to the highest tower, even, I suppose, the Campanile, and ride any horse, however wild. At the Bargello may be seen Alberti's portrait, on a medal designed by Pisanello. The old medals are indeed the best authority for the lineaments of the great men of the Renaissance, better far than paint. At South Kensington thousands may be seen, either in the original or in reproduction.

In the right aisle we saw Bernardo Rossellino's tomb of Leonardo Bruni; in the left is that of Bruni's successor as Secretary of State, Carlo Marsuppini, by Desiderio da Settignano, which is high among the most beautiful monuments that exist. "Faine, faine!" says Alfred Branconi, with his black eyes dimmed; and this though he has seen it every day for years and explained its beauties in the same words. Everything about it is beautiful, as the photograph which I give in this volume will help the reader to believe: proportions, figures, and tracery; but I still consider Mino's monument to Ugo in the Badia the finest Florentine example of the gentler memorial style, as contrasted with the severe Michelangelesque manner. Mino, it must be remembered, was Desiderio's pupil, as Desiderio was Donatello's. Note how Desiderio, by an inspiration, opened the leaf-work at each side of the sarcophagus and instantly the great solid mass of marble became light, almost buoyant. Never can a few strokes of the chisel have had so transforming an effect. There is some doubt as to whether the boys are just where the sculptor set them, and the upper ones with their garlands are thought to be a later addition; but we are never likely to know. The returned visitor from Florence will like to be reminded that, as of so many others of the best Florentine sculptures, there is a cast of this at South Kensington.

The last tomb of the highest importance in the church is that of Galileo, the astronomer, who died in 1642; but it is not interesting as a work of art. In the centre of the church is a floor-tomb by Ghiberti, with a bronze figure of a famous Franciscan, Francesco Sansoni da Brescia.

Next the sacristy. Italian priests apparently have no resentment against inquisitive foreigners who are led into their dressing-rooms while sumptuous and significant vestments are being donned; but I must confess to feeling it for them, and if my impressions of the S. Croce sacristy are meagre and confused it is because of a certain delicacy that I experienced in intruding upon their rites. For on both occasions when I visited the sacristy there were several priests either robing or disrobing. Apart from a natural disinclination to invade privacy, I am so poor a Roman Catholic as to be in some doubt as to whether one has a right to be so near such a mystery at all. But I recollect that in this sacristy are treasures of wood and iron–the most beautiful intarsia wainscotting I ever saw, by Giovanni di Michele, with a frieze of wolves and foliage, and fourteenth-century iron gates to the little chapel, pure Gothic in design, with a little rose window at the top, delicate beyond words: all which things once again turn the thoughts to this wonderful Italy of the fourteenth and fifteenth century, when not even the best was good enough for those who built churches, but something miraculous was demanded from every craftsman.

At the end of the passage in which the sacristy is situated is the exquisite little Cappella Medici, which Michelozzo, the architect of S. Marco and the Palazzo Medici, and for a while Donatello's partner, built for his friend Cosimo de' Medici, who though a Dominican in his cell at S. Marco was a Franciscan here, but by being equally a patron dissociated himself from partisanship. Three treasures in particular does this little temple hold: Giotto's "Coronation of the Virgin"; the della Robbia altar relief, and Mino da Fiesole's tabernacle. Giotto's picture, which is signed, once stood as altar-piece in the Baroncelli chapel of the church proper. In addition to the beautiful della Robbia altar-piece, so happy and holy–which Alfred Branconi boldly calls Luca–there is over the door Christ between two angels, a lovely example of the same art. For a subtler, more modern and less religious mind, we have but to turn to the tabernacle by Mino, every inch of which is exquisite.

On the same wall is a curious thing. In the eighteen-sixties died a Signor Lombardi, who owned certain reliefs which he believed to be Donatello's. When his monument was made these ancient works were built into them and here and there gilded (for it is a wicked world and there was no taste at that time). One's impulse is not to look at this encroaching piece of novelty at all; but one should resist that feeling, because, on examination, the Madonna and Children above Signor Lombardi's head become exceedingly interesting. Her hands are the work of a great artist, and they are really holding the Child. Why this should not be an early Donatello I do not see.

The cloisters of S. Croce are entered from the piazza, just to the right of the church: the first, a little ornate, by Arnolfo, and the second, until recently used as a barracks but now being restored to a more pacific end, by Brunelleschi, and among the most perfect of his works. Brunelleschi is also the designer of the Pazzi chapel in the first cloisters. The severity of the façade is delightfully softened and enlivened by a frieze of mischievous cherubs' heads, the joint work of Donatello and Desiderio. Donatello's are on the right, and one sees at once that his was the bolder, stronger hand. Look particularly at the laughing head fourth from the right. But that one of Desiderio's over the middle columns has much charm and power. The doors, from Brunelleschi's own hand, in a doorway perfect in scale, are noble and worthy. The chapel itself I find too severe and a little fretted by its della Robbias and the multiplicity of circles. It is called Brunelleschi's masterpiece, but I prefer both the Badia of Fiesole and the Old Sacristy at S. Lorenzo, and I remember with more pleasure the beautiful doorway leading from the Arnolfo cloisters to the Brunelleschi cloisters, which probably is his too. The della Robbia reliefs, once one can forgive them for being here, are worth study. Nothing could be more charming (or less conducive to a methodical literary morning) than the angel who holds S. Matthew's ink-pot. But I think my favourite of all is the pensive apostle who leans his cheek on his hand and his elbow on his book. This figure alone proves what a sculptor Luca was, apart altogether from the charm of his mind and the fascination of his chosen medium.

This chapel was once the scene of a gruesome ceremony. Old Jacopo Pazzi, the head of the family at the time of the Pazzi conspiracy against the Medici, after being hanged from a window of the Palazzo Vecchio, was buried here. Some short while afterwards Florence was inundated by rain to such an extent that the vengeance of God was inferred, and, casting about for a reason, the Florentines decided that it was because Jacopo had been allowed to rest in sacred soil. A mob therefore rushed to S. Croce, broke open his tomb and dragged his body through the streets, stopping on their way at the Pazzi palace to knock on the door with his skull. He was then thrown into the swollen Arno and borne away by the tide.

In the old refectory of the convent are now a number of pictures and fragments of sculpture. The "Last Supper," by Taddeo Gaddi, on the wall, is notable for depicting Judas, who had no shrift at the hands of the painters, without a halo. Castagno and Ghirlandaio, as we shall see, under similar circumstances, placed him on the wrong side of the table. In either case, but particularly perhaps in Taddeo's picture, the answer to Christ's question, which Leonardo at Milan makes so dramatic, is a foregone conclusion. The "Crucifixion" on the end wall, at the left, is interesting as having been painted for the Porta S. Gallo (in the Piazza Cavour) and removed here. All the gates of Florence had religious frescoes in them, some of which still remain. The great bronze bishop is said to be by Donatello and to have been meant for Or San Michele; but one does not much mind.

One finds occasion to say so many hard things of the Florentine disregard of ancient art that it is peculiarly a pleasure to see the progress that is being made in restoring Brunelleschi's perfect cloisters at S. Croce to their original form. When they were turned into barracks the Loggia was walled in all round and made into a series of rooms. These walls are now gradually coming away, the lovely pillars being again isolated, the chimneys removed, and everything lightly washed. Grass has also been sown in the great central square. The crumbling of the decorative medals in the spandrels of the cloisters cannot of course be restored; but one does not complain of such natural decay as that.

CHAPTER XVI

THE Accademia

Michelangelo–The David–The tomb of Julius–A contrast–Fra Angelico–The beatific painter–Cimabue and Giotto–Masaccio–Gentile da Fabriano–Domenico Ghirlandaio–Fra Angelico again–Fra Bartolommeo–Perugino–Botticelli–The "Primavera"–Leonardo da Vinci and Verrocchio–Botticelli's sacred pictures–Botticini–Tapestries of Eden.

The Accademia delle Belle Arti is in the Via Ricasoli, that street which seen from the top of the Campanile is the straightest thing in Florence, running like a ruled line from the Duomo to the valley of the Mugnone. Upstairs are modern painters: but upstairs I have never been. It is the ground-floor rooms that are so memorable, containing as they do a small but very choice collection of pictures illustrating the growth of Italian art, with particular emphasis on Florentine art; the best assemblage of the work of Fra Angelico that exists; and a large gallery given up to Michelangelo's sculpture: originals and casts. The principal magnets that draw people here, no doubt, are the Fra Angelicos and Botticelli's "Primavera"; but in five at least of the rooms there is not an uninteresting picture, while the collection is so small that one can study it without fatigue–no little matter after the crowded Uffizi and

Pitti.

It is a simple matter to choose in such a book as this the best place in which to tell something of the life-story of, say, Giotto and Brunelleschi and the della Robbias; for at a certain point their genius is found concentrated–Donatello's and the della Robbias' in the Bargello and those others at the Duomo and Campanile. But with Michelangelo it is different, he is so distributed over the city–his gigantic David here, the Medici tombs at S. Lorenzo, his fortifications at S. Miniato, his tomb at S. Croce, while there remains his house as a natural focus of all his activities. I have, however, chosen the Medici chapel as the spot best suited for his biography, and therefore will here dwell only on the originals that are preserved about the David. The David himself, superb and confident, is the first thing you see in entering the doors of the gallery. He stands at the end, white and glorious, with his eyes steadfastly measuring his antagonist and calculating upon what will be his next move if the sling misdirects the stone. Of the objection to the statue as being not representative of the Biblical figure I have said something in the chapter on the Bargello, where several Davids come under review. Yet, after all that can be said against its dramatic fitness, the statue remains an impressive and majestic yet strangely human thing. There it is–a sign of what a little Italian sculptor with a broken nose could fashion with his mallet and chisel from a mass of marble four hundred and more years ago.

Its history is curious. In 1501, when Michelangelo was twenty-six and had just returned to Florence from Rome with a great reputation as a sculptor, the joint authorities of the cathedral and the Arte della Lana offered him a huge block of marble that had been in their possession for thirty-five years, having been worked upon clumsily by a sculptor named Baccellino and then set aside. Michelangelo was told that if he accepted it he must carve from it a David and have it done in two years. He began in September, 1501, and finished in January, 1504, and a committee was appointed to decide upon its position, among them being Leonardo da Vinci, Perugino, Lorenzo di Credi, Filippino Lippi, Botticelli, and Andrea della Robbia,

There were three suggested sites: the Loggia de' Lanzi; the courtyard of the Palazzo Vecchio, where Verrocchio's little boudoir David then stood (now in the Bargello) and where his Cupid and dolphin now are; and the place where it now stands, then occupied by Donatello's Judith and Holofernes. This last was finally selected, not by the committee but by the determination of Michelangelo himself, and Judith and Holofernes were moved to the Loggia de' Lanzi to their present position. The David was set up in May, 1504, and remained there for three hundred and sixty-nine years, suffering no harm from the weather but having an arm broken in the Medici riots in 1527. In 1878, however, it was decided that further exposure might be injurious, and so the statue was moved here to its frigid niche and a replica in marble afterwards set up in its place. Since this glorious figure is to be seen thrice in Florence, he may be said to have become the second symbol of the city, next the fleur-de-lis.

The Tribuna del David, as the Michelangelo salon is called, has among other originals several figures intended for that tomb of Pope Julius II (whose portrait by Raphael we have seen at the Uffizi) which was to be the eighth wonder of the world, and by which the last years of the sculptor's life were rendered so unhappy. The story is a miserable one. Of the various component parts of the tomb, finished or unfinished, the best known is the Moses at S. Pietro in Vincoli at Rome, reproduced in plaster here, in the Accademia, beneath the bronze head of its author. Various other parts are in Rome too; others here; one or two may be at the Bargello (although some authorities give these supposed Michelangelos to Vincenzo Danti); others are in the grotto of the Boboli Gardens; and the Louvre has what is in some respects the finest of the "Prisoners".

The first statue on the right of the entrance of the Tribuna del David is a group called "Genio Vittorioso". Here in the old man we see rock actually turned to life; in the various "Prisoners" near we see life emerging from rock; in the David we forget the rock altogether. One wonders how Michelangelo went to work. Did the shape of the block of marble influence him, or did he with his mind's eye, the Röntgen rays of genius, see the figure within it, embedded in the midst, and hew and chip until it disclosed? On the back of the fourth statue on the left a monkish face has been incised: probably some visitor to the studio. After looking at these originals and casts, and remembering those other Michelangelo sculptures elsewhere in Florence–the tombs of the Medici, the Brutus and the smaller David–turn to the bronze head over the cast of Moses and reflect upon the author of it all: the profoundly sorrowful eyes behind which so much power and ambition and disappointment dwelt.

It is peculiarly interesting to walk out of the Michelangelo gallery into the little room containing the Fra Angelicos: to pass from a great melancholy saturnine sculptor, the victim of the caprice of princes temporal and spiritual, his eyes troubled with world knowledge and world weariness, to the childlike celebrant of the joy of simple faith who painted these gay and happy pictures. Fra Angelico–the sweetest of all the Florentine painters–was a monk of Fiesole, whose real name was Guido Petri da Mugello, but becoming a Dominican he called himself Giovanni, and now through the sanctity and happiness of his brush is for all time Beato Angelico. He was born in 1390, nearly sixty years after Giotto's death, when Chaucer was fifty, and Richard II on the English throne. His early years were spent in exile from Fiesole, the brothers having come into difficulties with the Archbishop, but by 1418 he was again at Fiesole, and when in 1436 Cosimo de' Medici, returned from exile at Venice, set his friend Michelozzo upon building the convent of S. Marco, Fra Angelico was fetched from Fiesole to decorate the walls. There, and here, in the Accademia, are his chief works assembled; but he worked also at Fiesole, at Cortona, and at Rome, where he painted frescoes in the chapel of Nicholas V in the Vatican and where he died, aged sixty-eight, and was buried. It was while at Rome that the Pope offered him the priorship of S. Marco, which he declined as being unworthy, but recommended Antonio, "the good archbishop".–That practically is his whole life. As to his character, let Vasari tell us. "He would often say that whosoever practised art needed a quiet life and freedom from care, and he who occupies himself with the things of Christ ought always to be with Christ. . . . Some say that Fra Giovanni never took up his brush without first making a prayer. . . . He never made a crucifix when the tears did not course down his cheeks." The one curious thing–to me–about Fra Angelico is that he has not been canonized. If ever a son of the Church toiled for her honour and for the happiness of mankind it was he.

There are examples of Fra Angelico's work elsewhere in Florence; the large picture in Room I of this gallery; the large altar-piece at the Uffizi, with certain others; the series of mural paintings in the cells of S. Marco; and his pictures will be found not only elsewhere in Florence and Italy but in the chief galleries of the world; for he was very assiduous. We have an excellent example at the National Gallery, No. 663; but this little room gives us the artist and rhapsodist most completely. In looking at his pictures, three things in particular strike the mind: the skill with which he composed them; his mastery of light; and–and here he is unique–the pleasure he must have had in painting them. All seem to have been play; he enjoyed the toil exactly as a child enjoys the labour of building a house with toy bricks. Nor, one feels, could he be depressed. Even in his Crucifixions there is a certain underlying happiness, due to his knowledge that the Crucified was to rise again and ascend to Heaven and enjoy eternal felicity. Knowing this (as he did know it) how could he be wholly cast down? You see it again in the Flagellation of Christ, in the series of six scenes (No. 237). The scourging is almost a festival. But best of all I like the Flight into Egypt, in No. 235. Everything here is joyous and (in spite of the terrible cause of the journey) bathed in the sunny light of the age of innocence: the landscape; Joseph, younger than usual, brave and resolute and undismayed by the curious turn in his fortunes; and Mary with the child in her arms, happy and pretty, seated securely on an amiable donkey that has neither bit nor bridle. It is when one looks at Fra Angelico that one understands how wise were the Old Masters to seek their inspiration in the life of Christ. One cannot imagine Fra Angelico's existence in a pagan country. Look, in No. 236, at the six radiant and rapturous angels clustering above the manger. Was there ever anything prettier? But I am not sure that I do not most covet No. 250, Christ crucified and two saints, and No. 251, the Coronation of the Virgin, for their beauty of light.

In the photographs No. 246–a Deposition–is unusually striking, but in the original, although beautiful, it is far less radiant than usual with this painter. It has, however, such feeling as to make it especially memorable among the many treatments of this subject. What is generally considered the most important work in this room is the Last Judgment, which is certainly extraordinarily interesting, and in the hierarchy of heaven and the company of the blest Fra Angelico is in a very acceptable mood. The benignant Christ Who divides the sheep and the goats; the healthy ripe-lipped Saints and Fathers who assist at the tribunal and have never a line of age or experience on their blooming cheeks; the monks and nuns, just risen from their graves, who embrace each other in the meads of paradise with such fervour–these have much of the charm of little flowers. But in delineating the damned the painter is in strange country. It was a subject of which he knew nothing, and the introduction among them of monks of the rival order of S. Francis is mere party politics and a blot.

There are two other rooms here, but Fra Angelico spoils us for them. Four panels by another Frate, but less radiant, Lippo Lippi, are remarkable, particularly the figure of the Virgin in the Annunciation; and there is a curious series of scenes entitled "L'Albero della Croce," by an Ignoto of the fourteenth century, with a Christ crucified in the midst and all Scripture in medallions around him, the tragedy of Adam and Eve at the foot (mutilated by some chaste pedant) being very quaint. And in Angelico's rooms there is a little, modest Annunciation by one of his school–No. 256–which shows what a good influence he was, and to which the eye returns and returns. Here also, on easels, are two portraits of Vallombrosan monks by Fra Bartolommeo, serene, and very sympathetically painted, which cause one to regret the deterioration in Italian ecclesiastic physiognomy; and Andrea del

Sarto's two pretty angels, which one so often finds in reproduction, are here too.

Let us now enter the first room of the collection proper and begin at the very beginning of Tuscan art, for this collection is historical and not fortuitous like that of the Pitti. The student may here trace the progress of Tuscan painting from the level to the highest peaks and downwards again. The Accademia was established with this purpose by that enlightened prince, Peter Leopold, Grand Duke of Tuscany, in 1784. Other pictures not wholly within his scheme have been added since, together with the Michelangelo statues and casts; but they do not impair the original idea. For the serious student the first room is of far the most importance, for there he may begin with Cimabue (? 1240-? 1302), and Giotto (1267-? 1337), and pass steadily to Luca Signorelli (? 1450-1523). For the most part the pictures in this room appeal to the inquirer rather than the sightseer; but there is not one that is without interest, while three works of extraordinary charm have thoughtfully been enisled, on screens, for special attention–a Fra Angelico, a Fabriano, and a Ghirlandaio. Before reaching these, let us look at the walls.

The first large picture, on the left, the Cimabue, marks the transition from Byzantine art to Italian art. Giovanni Cimabue, who was to be the forerunner of the new art, was born about 1240. At that time there was plenty of painting in Italy, but it was Greek, the work of artists at Constantinople (Byzantium), the centre of Christianity in the eastern half of the Roman Empire and the fount of ecclesiastical energy, and it was crude workmanship, existing purely as an accessory of worship. Cimabue, of whom, I may say, almost nothing definite is known, and upon whom the delightful but casual old Vasari is the earliest authority, as Dante was his first eulogist, carried on the Byzantine tradition, but breathed a little life into it. In his picture here we see him feeling his way from the unemotional painted symbols of the Faith to humanity itself. One can understand this large panel being carried (as we know the similar one at S. Maria Novella was) in procession and worshipped, but it is nearer to the icon of the Russian peasant of today than to a Raphael. The Madonna is above life; the Child is a little man. This was painted, say, in 1280, as an altar-piece for the Badia of S. Trinità at Florence.

Next came Giotto, Cimabue's pupil, born about 1267, whom we have met already as an architect, philosopher, and innovator; and in the second picture in this room, from Giotto's brush, we see life really awakening. The Madonna is vivifying; the Child is nearer childhood; we can believe that here are veins with blood in them. Moreover, whereas Cimabue's angels brought masonry, these bring flowers. It is crude, no doubt, but it is enough; the new art, which was to counterfeit and even extend nature, has really begun; the mystery and glory of painting are assured and the door opened for Botticelli.

But much had to happen first, particularly the mastery of the laws of perspective, and it was not (as we have seen) until Ghiberti had got to work on his first doors, and Brunelleschi was studying architecture and Uccello sitting up all night at his desk, that painting as we know it–painting of men and women "in the round"–could be done, and it was left for a youth who was not born until Giotto had been dead sixty-four years to do this first as a master–one Tommaso di Ser Giovanni Guido da Castel San Giovanni, known as Masaccio, or Big Tom. The three great names then in the evolution of Italian painting, a subject to which I return in chapter XXV, on the Carmine, are Cimabue, Giotto, Masaccio.

We pass on at the Accademia from Cimabue's pupil Giotto, to Giotto's followers, Taddeo Gaddi and Bernardo Daddi, and Daddi's follower Spinello Aretino, and the long dependent and interdependent line of painters. For the most part they painted altar-pieces, these early craftsmen, the Church being the principal patron of art. These works are many of them faded and so elementary as to have but an antiquarian interest; but think of the excitement in those days when the picture was at last ready, and, gay in its gold, was erected in the chapel! Among the purely ecclesiastical works No. 137, an Annunciation by Giovanni del Biondo (second half of the fourteenth century), is light and cheerful, and No. 142, the Crowning of the Virgin, by Rosello di Jacopo Franchi (1376-1456), has some delightful details and is everywhere joyous, with a charming green pattern in it. The wedding scenes in No. 147 give us Florentine life on the mundane side with some valuable thoroughness, and the Pietro Lorenzetti above–scenes in the life of S. Umilita–is very quaint and cheery and was painted as early as 1316. The little Virgin adoring, No. 160, in the corner, by the fertile Ignoto, is charmingly pretty.

And now for the three screens, notable among the screens of the galleries of Europe as holding three of the happiest pictures ever painted. The first is the Adoration of the Magi, by Gentile da Fabriano, an artist of whom one sees too little. His full name was Gentile di Niccolò di Giovanni Massi, and he was born at Fabriano between 1360 and 1370, some twenty years before Fra Angelico. According to Vasari he was Fra Angelico's master, but that is now considered doubtful, and yet the three little scenes from the life of Christ in the predella of this picture are nearer Fra Angelico in spirit and charm than any, not by a follower, that I have seen. Gentile did much work at Venice before he came to Florence, in 1422, and this picture, which is considered his masterpiece, was painted in 1423 for S. Trinita. He died four years later. Gentile was charming rather than great, and to this work might be applied Ruskin's sarcastic description of poor Ghirlandaio's frescoes, that they are mere goldsmith's work; and yet it is much more, for it has gaiety and sweetness and the nice thoughtfulness that made the Child a real child, interested like a child in the bald head of the kneeling mage; while the predella is not to be excelled in its modest, tender beauty by any in Florence; and predellas, I may remark again, should never be overlooked, strong as the tendency is to miss them. Many a painter has failed in the large space or made only a perfunctory success, but in the small has achieved real feeling. Gentile's Holy Family on its way to Egypt is never to be forgotten. Not so radiant as Fra Angelico's, in the room we have visited out of due course, but as charming in its own manner–both in personages and landscape; while the city to which Joseph leads the donkey (again without reins) is the most perfect thing out of fairyland.

Ghirlandaio's picture, which is the neighbour of Gentile's, is as a whole nearer life and one of his most attractive works. It is, I think, excelled only by his very similar Adoration of the Magi at the Spedale degli Innocenti, which, however, it is difficult to see; and it is far beyond the examples at the Uffizi, which are too hot. Of the life of this artist, who was Michelangelo's master, I shall speak in the chapter on S. Maria Novella. This picture, which represents the Adoration of the Shepherds, was painted in 1485, when the artist was thirty-six. It is essentially pleasant: a religious picture on the sunny side. The Child is the soul of babyish content, equally amused with its thumb and the homage it is receiving. Close by is a goldfinch unafraid; in the distance is a citied valley, with a river winding in it; and down a neighbouring hill, on the top of which the shepherds feed their flocks, comes the imposing procession of the Magi. Joseph is more than commonly perplexed, and the disparity between his own and his wife's age, which the old masters agreed to make considerable, is more considerable than usual.

Both Gentile and Ghirlandaio chose a happy subject and made it happier; Fra Angelico (for the third screen picture) chose a melancholy subject and made it happy, not because that was his intention, but because he could not help it. He had only one set of colours and one set of countenances, and since the colours were of the gayest and the countenances of the serenest, the result was bound to be peaceful and glad. This picture is a large "Deposizione della Croce," an altar piece for S. Trinità. There is such joy in the painting and light in the sky that a child would clap his hands at it all, and not least at the vermilion of the Redeemer's blood. Fra Angelico gave thought to every touch: and his beatific holiness floods the work. Each of these three great pictures, I may add, has its original frame.

The room which leads from this one is much less valuable; but Fra Bartolommeo's Vision of S. Bernard has lately been brought to an easel here to give it character. I find this the Frate's most beautiful work. It may have details that are a little crude, and the pointed nose of the Virgin is not perhaps in accordance with the best tradition, while she is too real for an apparition; but the figure of the kneeling saint is masterly and the landscape lovely in subject and feeling. Here too is Fra Bartolommeo's portrait of Savonarola, in which the reformer is shown as personating S. Peter Martyr. The picture was not painted from life, but from an earlier portrait. Fra Bartolommeo had some reason to know what Savonarola was like, for he was his personal friend and a brother in the same convent of S. Marco, a few yards from the Accademia, across the square. He was born in 1475 and was apprenticed to the painter Cosimo Rosselli; but he learned more from studying Masaccio's frescoes at the Carmine and the work of Leonardo da Vinci. It was in 1495 that he came under the influence of Savonarola, and he was the first artist to run home and burn his studies from the nude in response to the preacher's denunciations. Three years later, when Savonarola was an object of hatred and the convent of S. Marco was besieged, the artist was with him, and he then made a vow that if he lived he would join the order; and this promise he kept, although not until Savonarola had been executed. For a while, as a monk, he laid aside the brush, but in 1506 he resumed it and painted until his death, in 1517. He was buried at S. Marco.

In his less regenerate days Fra Bartolommeo's greatest friend was the jovial Mariotto Albertinelli, whose rather theatrical Annunciation hangs between a number of the monk's other portraits, all very interesting. Of Albertinelli I have spoken earlier. Before leaving, look at the tiny Ignoto next the door–a Madonna and Child, the child eating a pomegranate. It is a little picture to steal.

In the next room are a number of the later and showy painters, such as Carlo Dolci, Lorenzo Lippi, and Francesco Furini, all bold, dashing, self-satisfied hands, in whom (so near the real thing) one can take no interest. Nothing to steal here.

Returning through Sala Prima we come to the Sala del Perugino and are among the masters once more–riper and richer than most of those we have already seen, for Tuscan art here reaches its finest flower. Perugino is here and Botticelli, Fra Bartolommeo and Leonardo, Luca Signorelli, Fra Lippo Lippi and Filippino Lippi. And here is a Masaccio. The great Perugino Assumption has all his mellow sunset calm, and never was a landscape more tenderly sympathetic. The same painter's Deposition hangs next, and the custodian brings a magnifying glass that the tears on the Magdalen's cheek may be more closely observed; but the third, No. 53, Christ in the Garden of Gethsemane, is finer, and here again the landscape and light are perfect. For the rest, there is a Royal Academy Andrea and a formal Ghirlandaio.

And now we come to Botticelli, who although less richly represented in numbers than at the Uffizi, is for the majority of his admirers more to be sought here, by reason of the "Primavera" allegory, which is the Accademia's most powerful magnet. The Botticellis are divided between two rooms, the "Primavera" being in the first. The first feeling one has is how much cooler it is here than among the Peruginos, and how much gayer; for not only is there the "Primavera," but Fra Lippo Lippi is here too, with a company of angels helping to crown the Virgin, and a very sweet, almost transparent, little Madonna adoring–No. 79–which one cannot forget.

The "Primavera" is not wearing too well: one sees that at once. Being in tempera it cannot be cleaned, and a dulness is overlaying it; but nothing can deprive the figure of Spring of her joy and movement, a floating type of conquering beauty and youth. The most wonderful thing about this wonderful picture is that it should have been painted when it was: that, suddenly, out of a solid phalanx of Madonnas should have stepped these radiant creatures of the joyous earth, earthy and joyful. And not only that they should have so surprisingly and suddenly emerged, but that after all these years this figure of Spring should still be the finest of her kind. That is the miracle! Luca Signorelli's flowers at the Uffizi remain the best, but Botticelli's are very thoughtful and before the grass turned black they must have been very lovely; the exquisite drawing of the irises in the right-hand corner can still be traced, although the colour has gone. The effect now is rather like a Chinese painting. For the history of the "Primavera" and its signification, one must turn back to Chapter X.

I spoke just now of Luca's flowers. There are others in his picture in this room–botanist's flowers as distinguished from painter's flowers: the wild strawberry beautifully straggling. This picture is one of the most remarkable in all Florence to me: a Crucifixion to which the perishing of the colour has given an effect of extreme delicacy, while the group round the cross on the distant mound has a quality for which one usually goes to Spanish art. The Magdalen is curiously sulky and human. Into the skull at the foot of the cross creeps a lizard.

This room has three Lippo Lippis, which is an interesting circumstance when we remember that that dissolute brother was the greatest influence on Botticelli. The largest is the Coronation of the Virgin with its many lilies–a picture which one must delight in, so happy and crowded is it, but which never seems to me quite what it should be. The most fascinating part of it is the figures in the two little medallions: two perfect pieces of colour and design. The kneeling monk on the right is Lippo Lippi himself. Near it is the Madonna adoring, No. 79, of which I have spoken, with herself so luminous and the background so dark; the other–No. 82–is less remarkable. No. 81, above it, is by Browning's Pacchiorotto (who worked in distemper); close by is the Masaccio, which has a deep, quiet beauty; and beneath it is a richly coloured predella by Andrea del Sarto, the work of a few hours, I should guess, and full of spirit and vigour. It consists of four scriptural scenes which might be called the direct forerunners of Sir John Gilbert and the modern illustrators. Lastly we have what is in many ways the most interesting picture in Florence–No. 71, the Baptism of Christ–for it is held by some authorities to be the only known painting by Verrocchio, whose sculptures we saw in the Bargello and at Or San Michele, while in one of the angels–that surely on the left–we are to see the hand of his pupil Leonardo da Vinci. Their faces are singularly sweet. Other authorities consider not only that Verrocchio painted the whole picture himself but that he painted also the Annunciation at the Uffizi to which Leonardo's name is given. Be that as it may–and we shall never know–this is a beautiful thing. According to Vasari it was the excellence of Leonardo's contribution which decided Verrocchio to give up the brush. Among the thoughts of Leonardo is one which comes to mind with peculiar force before this work when we know its story: "Poor is the pupil who does not surpass his master".

The second Sala di Botticelli has not the value of the first. It has magnificent examples of Botticelli's sacred work, but the other pictures are not the equal of those in the other rooms. Chief of the Botticellis is No. 85, "The Virgin and Child with divers Saints," in which there are certain annoying and restless elements. One feels that in the accessories–the flooring, the curtains, and gilt–the painter was wasting his time, while the Child is too big. Botticelli was seldom too happy with his babies. But the face of the Saint in green and blue on the left is most exquisitely painted, and the Virgin has rather less troubled beauty than usual. The whole effect is not quite spiritual, and the symbolism of the nails and the crown of thorns held up for the Child to see is rather too cruel and obvious. I like better the smaller picture with the same title–No. 88–in which the Saints at each side are wholly beautiful in Botticelli's wistful way, and the painting of their heads and head-dresses is so perfect as to fill one with a kind of despair. But taken altogether one must consider Botticelli's triumph in the Accademia to be pagan rather than sacred.

No. 8, called officially School of Verrocchio, and by one firm of photographers Botticini, and by another Botticelli, is a fine free thing, low in colour, with a quiet landscape, and is altogether a delight. It represents Tobias and the three angels, and Raphael moves nobly, although not with quite such a step as the radiant figure in a somewhat similar picture in our own National Gallery–No. 781–which, once confidently given to Verrocchio, is now attributed to Botticini; while our No. 296, which the visitor from Florence on returning to London should hasten to examine, is no longer Verrocchio but School of Verrocchio. When we think of these attributions and then look at No. 154 in the Accademia–another Tobias and the Angel, here given to Botticini–we have a concrete object lesson in the perilous career that awaits the art expert,

The other pictures here are two sunny panels by Ridolfo Ghirlandaio, high up, with nice easy colouring; No. 92, an Adoration of the Shepherds by Lorenzo di Credi, with a good landscape and all very sweet and quiet; No. 98, a Deposition by Filippino Lippi and Perugino, in collaboration, with very few signs of Filippino; and No. 90, a Resurrection by Raffaellino del Garbo, an uncommon painter in Florence; the whole thing a tour de force, but not important.

And now let us look at the Angelicos again.

Before leaving the Accademia for the last time, one should glance at the tapestries near the main entrance, just for fun. That one in which Adam names the animals is so delightfully naive that it ought to be reproduced as a nursery wall-paper. The creatures pass in review in four processions, and Adam must have had to be uncommonly quick to make up his mind first and then rattle out their resultant names in the time. The main procession is that of the larger quadrupeds, headed by the unicorn in single glory; and the moment chosen by the artist is that in which the elephant, having just heard his name (for the first time) and not altogether liking it, is turning towards Adam in surprised remonstrance. The second procession is of reptiles, led by the snail; the third, the smaller quadrupeds, led by four rats, followed desperately close (but of course under the white flag) by two cats; while the fourth–all sorts and conditions of birds–streams through the air. The others in this series are all delightful, not the least being that in which God, having finished His work, takes Adam's arm and flies with him over the earth to point out its merits.

CHAPTER XVII

TWO Monasteries and a Procession

The Certosa–A Company of Uncles–The Cells–Machiavelli–Impruneta–The della Robbias–Pontassieve–Pelago–Milton's simile–Vallombrosa–S. Gualberto–Prato and the Lippis–The Grassina Albergo–An American invasion–The Procession of the Dead Christ–My loss.

Everyone who merely visits Florence holds it a duty to bring home at least one flask of the Val d'Ema liqueur from the Carthusian monastery four or five miles distant from the city, not because that fiery distillation is peculiarly attractive but because the vessels which contain it are at once pretty decorations and evidences of travel and culture. They can be bought in Florence itself, it is true (at a shop at the corner of the Via de' Cerretani, close to the Baptistery), but the Certosa is far too interesting to miss, if one has time to spare from the city's own treasures. The trams start from the Mercato Nuovo and come along the Via dell' Arcivescovado to the Baptistery, and so to the Porta Romana and out into the hilly country. The ride is dull and rather tiresome, for there is much waiting at sidings, but the expedition becomes attractive immediately the tram is left. There is then a short walk, principally up the long narrow approach to the monastery gates, outside which, when I was there, was sitting a beggar at a stone table, waiting for the bowl of soup to which all who ask are entitled.

Passing within the courtyard you ring the bell on the right and enter the waiting hall, from which, in the course of time, when a sufficient party has been gathered, an elderly monk in a white robe leads you away. How many monks there may be, I cannot say; but of the few of whom I caught a glimpse, all were alike in the possession of white beards, and all suggested uncles in fancy dress. Ours spoke good French and was clearly a man of parts. Lulled by his soothing descriptions I passed in a kind of dream through this ancient abode of peace.

The Certosa dates from 1341 and was built and endowed by a wealthy merchant named Niccolo Acciaioli, after whom the Lungarno Acciaioli is named. The members of the family are still buried here, certain of the tombstones bearing dates of the present century. To-day it is little but a show place, the cells of the monks being mostly empty and the sale of the liqueur its principal reason for existence. But the monks who are left take a pride in their church, which is attributed to Orcagna, and its possessions, among which come first the relief monuments of early Acciaioli in the floor of one of the chapels–the founder's being perhaps also the work of Orcagna, while that of his son Lorenzo, who died in 1353, is attributed by our cicerone to Donatello, but by others to an unknown hand. It is certainly very beautiful. These tombs are the very reverse of those which we saw in S. Croce; for those bear the obliterating traces of centuries of footsteps, so that some are nearly flat with the stones, whereas these have been railed off for ever and have lost nothing. The other famous Certosa tomb is that of Cardinal Angelo Acciaioli, which, once given to Donatello, is now sometimes attributed to Giuliano di Sangallo and sometimes to his son Francesco.

The Certosa has a few good pictures, but it is as a monastery that it is most interesting: as one of the myriad lonely convents of Italy, which one sees so constantly from the train, perched among the Apennines, and did not expect ever to enter. The cloisters which surround the garden, in the centre of which is a well, and beneath which is the distillery, are very memorable, not only for their beauty but for the sixty and more medallions of saints and evangelists all round it by Giovanni della Robbia. Here the monks have sunned themselves, and here been buried, these five and a half centuries. One suite of rooms is shown, with its own little private garden and no striking discomfort except the hole in the wall by the bed, through which the sleeper is awakened. From its balcony one sees the Etna far below and hears the roar of a weir, and away in the distance is Florence with the Duomo and a third of Giotto's Campanile visible above the intervening hills.

Having shown you all the sights the monk leads you again to the entrance hall and bids you good-bye, with murmurs of surprise and a hint of reproach on discovering a coin in his hand, for which, however, none the less, he manages in the recesses of his robe to find a place; and you are then directed to the room where the liqueur, together with sweets and picture post-cards, is sold by another monk, assisted by a lay attendant, and the visit to the Certosa is over.

The tram that passes the Certosa continues to S. Casciano in the Chianti district (but much wine is called Chianti that never came from here), where there is a point of interest in the house to which Machiavelli retired in 1512, to give himself to literature and to live that wonderful double life–a peasant loafer by day in the fields and the village inn, and at night, dressed in his noblest clothes, the cold, sagacious mentor of the rulers of mankind. But at S. Casciano I did not stop.

And farther still one comes to the village of Impruneta, after climbing higher and higher, with lovely calm valleys on either side coloured by silver olive groves and vivid wheat and maize, and studded with white villas and villages and church towers. On the road every woman in every doorway plaits straw with rapid fingers just as if we were in Bedfordshire. Impruneta is famous for its new terra-cotta vessels and its ancient della Robbias. For in the church is some of Luca's most exquisite work–an altarpiece with a frieze of aerial angels under it, and a stately white saint on either side, and the loveliest decorated columns imaginable; while in an adjoining chapel is a Christ crucified mourned by the most dignified and melancholy of Magdalens. Andrea della Robbia is here too, and here also is a richly designed cantoria by Mino da Fiesole. The village is not in the regular programme of visitors, and Baedeker ignores it; hence perhaps the excitement which an arrival from Florence causes, for the children turn out in battalions. The church is very dirty, and so indeed is everything else; but no amount of grime can disguise the charm of the cloisters.

The Certosa is a mere half-hour from Florence, Impruneta an hour and a half; but Vallombrosa asks a long day. One can go by rail, changing at Sant' Ellero into the expensive rack-and-pinion car which climbs through the vineyards to a point near the summit, and has, since it was opened, brought to the mountain so many new residents, whose little villas cling to the western slopes among the lizards, and, in summer, are smitten unbearably by the sun. But the best way to visit the monastery and the groves is by road. A motor-car no doubt makes little of the journey; but a carriage and pair such as I chartered at Florence for forty-five lire has to be away before seven, and, allowing three hours on the top, is not back again until the same hour in the evening; and this, the ancient way, with the beat of eight hoofs in one's ears, is the right way.

For several miles the road and the river–the Arno–run side by side–and the railway close by too–through venerable villages whose inhabitants derive their living either from the soil or the water, and amid vineyards all the time. Here and there a white villa is seen, but for the most part this is peasants' district: one such villa on the left, before Pontassieve, having about it, and on each side of its drive, such cypresses as one seldom sees and only Gozzoli or Mr. Sargent could rightly paint, each in his own style. Not far beyond, in a scrap of meadow by the road, sat a girl knitting in the morning sun–with a placid glance at us as we rattled by; and ten hours later, when we rattled past again, there she still was, still knitting, in the evening sun, and again her quiet eyes were just raised and dropped.

At Pontassieve we stopped a while for coffee at an inn at the corner of the square of pollarded limes, and while it was preparing watched the little crumbling town at work, particularly the cooper opposite, who was finishing a massive cask within whose recesses good Chianti is doubtless now maturing; and then on the white road again, to the turning, a mile farther on, to the left, where one bids the Arno farewell till the late afternoon. Steady climbing now, and then a turn to the right and we see Pelago before us, perched on its crags, and by and by come to it–a tiny town, with a clean and alluring inn, very different from the squalor of Pontassieve: famous in art and particularly Florentine art as being the birthplace of Lorenzo Ghiberti, who made the Baptistery doors. From Pelago the road descends with extreme steepness to a brook in a rocky valley, at a bridge over which the real climb begins, to go steadily on (save for another swift drop before Tosi) until Vallombrosa is reached, winding through woods all the way, chiefly chestnut–those woods which gave Milton, who was here in 1638, his famous simile. [6] The heat was now becoming intense (it was mid-September) and the horses were suffering, and most of this last stage was done at walking pace; but such was the exhilaration of the air, such the delight of the aromas which the breeze continually wafted from the woods, now sweet, now pungent, and always refreshing, that one felt no fatigue even though walking too. And so at last the monastery, and what was at that moment better than anything, lunch.

The beauty and joy of Vallombrosa, I may say at once, are Nature's, not man's. The monastery, which is now a Government school of forestry, is ugly and unkempt; the hotel is unattractive; the few people one meets want to sell something or take you for a drive. But in an instant in any direction one can be in the woods–and at this level they are pine woods, soft underfoot and richly perfumed–and a quarter of an hour's walking brings the view. It is then that you realize you are on a mountain indeed. Florence is to the north-west in the long Arno valley, which is here precipitous and narrow. The river is far below–if you slipped you would slide into it–fed by tumbling Apennine streams from both walls. The top of the mountain is heathery like

Scotland, and open; but not long will it be so, for everywhere are the fenced parallelograms which indicate that a villa is to be erected. Nothing, however, can change the mountain air or the glory of the surrounding heights.

Another view, unbroken by villas but including the monastery and the Foresters' Hotel in the immediate foreground, and extending as far as Florence itself (on suitable days), is obtained from Il Paradisino, a white building on a ledge which one sees from the hotel above the monastery. But that is not by any means the top. The view covers much of the way by which we came hither.

Of the monastery of Vallombrosa we have had foreshadowings in Florence. We saw at the Accademia two exquisite portraits by Fra Bartolommeo of Vallombrosan monks. We saw at the Bargello the remains of a wonderful frieze by Benedetto da Rovezzano for the tomb of the founder of the order, S. Giovanni Gualberto; we shall see at S. Miniato scenes in the saint's life on the site of the ancient chapel where the crucifix bent and blessed him. As the head of the monastery Gualberto was famous for the severity and thoroughness of his discipline. But though a martinet as an abbot, personally he was humble and mild. His advice on all kinds of matters is said to have been invited even by kings and popes. He invented the system of lay brothers to help with the domestic work of the convent; and after a life of holiness, which comprised several miracles, he died in 1073 and was subsequently canonized.

The monastery, as I have said, is now secularized, save for the chapel, where three resident monks perform service. One may wander through its rooms and see in the refectory, beneath portraits of famous brothers, the tables now laid for young foresters. The museum of forestry is interesting to those interested in museums of forestry.

It was to the monastery at Vallombrosa that the Brownings travelled in 1848 when Mrs. Browning was ill. But the abbot could not break the rules in regard to women, and after five days they had to return to Florence. Browning used to play the organ in the chapel, as, it is said, Milton had done two centuries earlier.

At such a height and with only a short season the hotel proprietors must do what they can, and prices do not rule low. A departing American was eyeing his bill with a rueful glance as we were leaving. "Milton had it wrong," he said to me (with the freemasonry of the plucked, for I knew him not), "what he meant was, 'thick as thieves'."

We returned by way of Sant' Ellero, the gallant horses trotting steadily down the hill, and then beside the Arno once more all the way to Florence. It chanced to be a great day in the city–September 20th, the anniversary of the final defeat of papal temporal power, in 1870–which we were not sorry to have missed, the first tidings coming to us from the beautiful tower of the Palazzo Vecchio which in honour of the occasion had been picked out with fairy lamps.

Among the excursions which I think ought to be made if one is in Florence for a justifying length of time is a visit to Prato. This ancient town one should see for several things: for its age and for its walls; for its great piazza (with a pile of vividly dyed yarn in the midst) surrounded by arches under which coppersmiths hammer all day at shining rotund vessels, while their wives plait straw; for Filippino Lippi's exquisite Madonna in a little mural shrine at the narrow end of the piazza, which a woman (fetched by a crowd of ragged boys) will unlock for threepence; and for the cathedral, with Filippino's dissolute father's frescoes in it, the Salome being one of the most interesting pre-Botticelli scenes in Italian art. If only it had its colour what a wonder of lightness and beauty this still would be! But probably most people are attracted to Prato chiefly by Donatello and Michelozzo's outdoor pulpit, the frieze of which is a kind of prentice work for the famous cantoria in the museum of the cathedral at Florence, with just such wanton boys dancing round it.

On Good Friday evening in the lovely dying April light I paid thirty centimes to be taken by tram to Grassina to see the famous procession of the Gesù Morto. The number of people on the same errand having thrown out the tram service, we had very long waits, while the road was thronged with other vehicles; and the result was I was tired enough–having been standing all the way–when Grassina was reached, for festivals six miles out of Florence at seven in the evening disarrange good habits. But a few pence spent in the albergo on bread and cheese and wine soon restored me. A queer cavern of a place, this inn, with rough tables, rows and rows of wine flasks, and an open fire behind the bar, tended by an old woman, from which everything good to eat proceeded rapidly without dismay–roast chicken and fish in particular. A strapping girl with high cheek bones and a broad dark comely face washed plates and glasses assiduously, and two waiters, with eyes as near together as monkeys', served the customers with bewildering intelligence. It was the sort of inn that in England would throw up its hands if you asked even for cold beef.

The piazza of Grassina, which, although merely a village, is enterprising enough to have a cinematoscope hall, was full of stalls given chiefly to the preparation and sale of cake like the Dutch wafelen, and among the stalls were conjurors, cheap-jacks, singers, and dice throwers; while every moment brought its fresh motor-car or carriage load, nearly all speaking English with a nasal twang. Meanwhile every one shouted, the naphtha flared, the drums beat, the horses champed. The street was full too, chiefly of peasants, but among them myriad resolute American virgins, in motor veils, whom nothing can ever surprise; a few American men, sceptical, as ever, of anything ever happening; here and there a diffident Englishwoman and Englishman, more in the background, but destined in the end to see all. But what I chiefly noticed was the native girls, with their proud bosoms carried high and nothing on their heads. They at any rate know their own future. No rushing over the globe for them, but the simple natural home life and children.

In the gloom the younger girls in white muslin were like pretty ghosts, each followed by a solicitous mother giving a touch here and a touch there–mothers who once wore muslin too, will wear it no more, and are now happy in pride in their daughters. And very little girls too–mere tots–wearing wings, who very soon were to join the procession as angels.

And all the while the darkness was growing, and on the hill where the church stands lights were beginning to move about, in that mysterious way which torches have when a procession is being mobilized, while all the villas on the hills around had their rows of candles.

And then the shifting flames came gradually into a mass and took a steady upward progress, and the melancholy strains of an ancient ecclesiastical lamentation reached our listening ears. As the lights drew nearer I left the bank where all the Mamies and Sadies with their Mommas were stationed and walked down into the river valley to meet the vanguard. On the bridge I found a little band of Roman soldiers on horseback, without stirrups, and had a few words with one of them as to his anachronistic cigarette, and then the first torches arrived, carried by proud little boys in red; and after the torches the little girls in muslin veils, which were, however, for the most part disarranged for the better recognition of relations and even more perhaps for recognition by relations: and very pretty this recognition was on both sides. And then the village priests in full canonicals, looking a little self-conscious; and after them the dead Christ on a litter carried by a dozen contadini who had a good deal to say to each other as they bore Him.

This was the same dead Christ which had been lying in state in the church, for the past few days, to be worshipped and kissed by the peasantry. I had seen a similar image at Settignano the day before and had watched how the men took it. They began by standing in groups in the piazza, gossipping. Then two or three would break away and make for the church. There, all among the women and children, half-shyly, half-defiantly, they pecked at the plaster flesh and returned to resume the conversation in the piazza with a new serenity and confidence in their hearts.

After the dead Christ came a triumphal car of the very little girls with wings, signifying I know not what, but intensely satisfying to the onlookers. One little wet-nosed cherub I patted, so chubby and innocent she was; and Heaven send that the impulse profited me! This car was drawn by an ancient white horse, amiable and tractable as a saint, but as bewildered as I as to the meaning of the whole strange business. After the car of angels a stalwart body of white-vestmented singers, sturdy fellows with black moustaches who had been all day among the vines, or steering placid white oxen through the furrows, and were now lifting their voices in a miserere. And after them the painted plaster Virgin, carried as upright as possible, and then more torches and the wailing band; and after the band another guard of Roman soldiers.

Such was the Grassina procession. It passed slowly and solemnly through the town from the hill and up the hill again; and not soon shall I forget the mournfulness of the music, which nothing of tawdriness in the constituents of the procession itself could rid of impressiveness and beauty. One thing is certain–all processions, by day or night, should first descend a hill and then ascend one. All should walk to melancholy strains. Indeed, a joyful procession becomes an impossible thought after this.

And then I sank luxuriously into a corner seat in the waiting tram, and, seeking for the return journey's thirty centimes, found that during the proceedings my purse had been stolen.

CHAPTER XVIII

S. Marco

Andrea del Castagno–"The Last Supper"–The stolen Madonna–Fra Angelico's frescoes–"Little Antony"–The good archbishop–The Buonuomini–Savonarola–The death of Lorenzo the Magnificent–Pope Alexander VI–The Ordeal by Fire–The execution–The S. Marco cells–The cloister frescoes–Ghirlandaio's "Last Supper"–Relics of old Florence–Pico and Politian–Piero di Cosimo–Andrea del Sarto.

From the Accademia it is but a step to S. Marco, across the Piazza, but it is well first to go a little beyond that in order to see a certain painting which both chronologically and as an influence comes before a painting that we shall find in the Museo S. Marco. We therefore cross the Piazza S. Marco to the Via d'Arrazzieri, which leads into the Via 27 Aprile, [7] where at a door on the left, marked A, is an ancient refectory, preserved as a picture gallery: the Cenacolo di S. Apollonia, all that is kept sacred of the monastery of S. Apollonia, now a military establishment. This room is important to students of art in containing so much work of Andrea del Castagno (1390-1457), to whom Vasari gives so black a character. The portrait frescoes are from the Villa Pandolfini (previously Carducci), and among them are Boccaccio, Petrarch, and Dante–who is here rather less ascetic than usual–none of whom the painter could have seen. There is also a very charming little cupid carrying a huge peacock plume. But "The Last Supper" is the glory of the room. This work, which belongs to the middle of the fifteenth century, is interesting as a real effort at psychology. Leonardo makes Judas leave his seat to ask if it is he that is meant–that being the dramatic moment chosen by this prince of painters: Castagno calls attention to Judas as an undesirable member of the little band of disciples by placing him apart, the only one on his side of the table; which was avoiding the real task, since naturally when one of the company was forced into so sinister a position the question would be already answered. Castagno indeed renders Judas so obviously untrustworthy as to make it a surprise that he ever was admitted among the disciples (or wished to be one) at all; while Vasari blandly suggests that he is the very image of the painter himself. Other positions which later artists converted into a convention may also be noted: John, for example, is reclining on the table in an ecstasy of affection and fidelity; while the Florentine loggia as the scene of the meal was often reproduced later.

Andrea del Castagno began life as a farm lad, but was educated as an artist at the cost of one of the less notable Medici. He had a vigorous way with his brush, as we see here and have seen elsewhere. In the Duomo, for example, we saw his equestrian portrait of Niccolò da Tolentino, a companion to Uccello's Hawkwood. When the Albizzi and Peruzzi intrigues which had led to the banishment of Cosimo de' Medici came to their final frustration with the triumphant return of Cosimo, it was Andrea who was commissioned by the Signoria to paint for the outside of the Bargello a picture of the leaders of the insurrection, upside down. Vasari is less to be trusted in his dates and facts in his memoir of Andrea del Castagno than anywhere else; for he states that he commemorated the failure of the Pazzi Conspiracy (which occurred twenty years after his death), and accuses him not only of murdering his fellow-painter Domenico Veneziano but confessing to the crime; the best answer to which allegation is that Domenico survived Andrea by four years.

We may now return to S. Marco. The convent as we now see it was built by Michelozzo, Donatello's friend and partner and the friend also of Cosimo de' Medici, at whose cost he worked here. Antonino, the saintly head of the monastery, having suggested to Cosimo that he should apply some of his wealth, not always too nicely obtained, to the Lord, Cosimo began literally to squander money on S. Marco, dividing his affection between S. Lorenzo, which he completed upon the lines laid down by his father, and this Dominican monastery, where he even had a cell reserved for his own use, with a bedroom in addition, whither he might now and again retire for spiritual refreshment and quiet.

It was at S. Marco that Cosimo kept the MSS. which he was constantly collecting, and which now, after curious vicissitudes, are lodged in Michelangelo's library at S. Lorenzo; and on his death he left them to the monks. Cosimo's librarian was Tommaso Parenticelli, a little busy man, who, to the general astonishment, on the death of Eugenius IV became Pope and took the name of Nicholas V. His energies as Pontiff went rather towards learning and art than anything else: he laid the foundations of the Vatican library, on the model of Cosimo's, and persuaded Fra Angelico to Rome to paint Vatican frescoes.

The magnets which draw every one who visits Florence to S. Marco are first Fra Angelico, and secondly Savonarola, or first Savonarola, and secondly Fra Angelico, according as one is constituted. Fra Angelico, at Cosimo's desire and cost, came from Fiesole to paint here; while Girolamo Savonarola, forced to leave Ferrara during the war, entered these walls in 1482. Fra Angelico in his single crucifixion picture in the first cloisters and in his great scene of the Mount of Olives in the chapter house shows himself less incapable of depicting unhappiness than we have yet seen him; but the most memorable of the ground-floor frescoes is the symbol of hospitality over the door of the wayfarers' room, where Christ is being welcomed by two Dominicans in the way that Dominicans (as contrasted with scoundrelly Franciscans) would of course welcome Him. In this Ospizio are three reliquaries which Fra Angelico painted for S. Maria Novella, now preserved here in a glass case. They represent the Madonna della Stella, the Coronation of the Virgin, and the Adoration of the Magi. All are in Angelico's happiest manner, with plenty of gold; and the predella of the Coronation is the prettiest thing possible, with its blue saints gathered about a blue Mary and Joseph, who bend over the Baby.

The Madonna della Stella is the picture which was stolen in 1911, but quickly recovered. It is part of the strange complexity of this world that it should equally contain artists such as Fra Angelico and thieves such as those who planned and carried out this robbery: nominally custodians of the museum. To repeat one of Vasari's sentences: "Some say that he never took up his brush without first making a prayer"....

The "Peter" with his finger to his lips, over the sacristy, is reminding the monks that that room is vowed to silence. In the chapter house is the large Crucifixion by the same gentle hand, his greatest work in Florence, and very fine and true in character. Beneath it are portraits of seventeen famous Dominicans with S. Dominic in the midst. Note the girl with the scroll in the right–how gay and light the colouring. Upstairs, in the cells, and preeminently in the passage, where his best known Annunciation is to be seen, Angelico is at his best. In each cell is a little fresco reminding the brother of the life of Christ–and of those by Angelico it may be said that each is as simple as it can be and as sweet: easy lines, easy colours, with the very spirit of holiness shining out. I think perhaps that the Coronation of the Virgin in the ninth cell, reproduced in this volume, is my favourite, as it is of many persons; but the Annunciation in the third, the two Maries at the Sepulchre in the eighth, and the Child in the Stable in the fifth, are ever memorable too. In the cell set apart for Cosimo de' Medici, No. 38, which the officials point out, is an Adoration of the Magi, painted there at Cosimo's express wish, that he might be reminded of the humility proper to rulers; and here we get one of the infrequent glimpses of this best and wisest of the Medici, for a portrait of him adorns it, with a wrong death-date on it.

Here also is a sensitive terra-cotta bust of S. Antonio, Cosimo's friend and another pride of the monastery: the monk who was also Archbishop of Florence until his death, and whom we saw, in stone, in a niche under the Uffizi. His cell was the thirty-first cell, opposite the entrance. This benign old man, who has one of the kindest faces of his time, which was often introduced into pictures, was appointed to the see at the suggestion of Fra Angelico, to whom Pope Eugenius (who consecrated the new S. Marco in 1442 and occupied Cosimo de' Medici's cell on his visit) had offered it; but the painter declined and put forward Antonio in his stead. Antonio Pierozzi, whose destiny it was to occupy this high post, to be a confidant of Cosimo de' Medici, and ultimately, in 1523, to be enrolled among the saints, was born at Florence in 1389. According to Butler, from the cradle "Antonino" or "Little Antony," as the Florentines affectionately called him, had "no inclination but to piety," and was an enemy even as an infant "both to sloth and to the amusements of children". As a schoolboy his only pleasure was to read the lives of the saints, converse with pious persons or to pray. When not at home or at school he was in church, either kneeling or lying prostrate before a crucifix, "with a perseverance that astonished everybody". S. Dominic himself, preaching at Fiesole, made him a Dominican, his answers to an examination of the whole decree of Gratian being the deciding cause, although Little Antony was then but sixteen. As a priest he was "never seen at the altar but bathed in tears". After being prior of a number of convents and a counsellor of much weight in convocation, he was made Archbishop of Florence: but was so anxious to avoid the honour and responsibility that he hid in the island of Sardinia. On being discovered he wrote a letter praying to be excused and watered it with his tears; but at last he consented and was consecrated in 1446.

As archbishop his life was a model of simplicity and solicitude. He thought only of his duties and the well-being of the poor. His purse was open to all in need, and he "often sold" his single mule in order to relieve some necessitous person. He gave up his garden to the growth of vegetables for the poor, and kept an ungrateful leper whose sores he dressed with his own hands. He died in 1459 and was canonized in 1523. His body was still free from corruption in 1559, when it was translated to the chapel in S. Marco prepared for it by the Salviati.

But perhaps the good Antonino's finest work was the foundation of a philanthropic society of Florentines which still carries on its good work. Antonino's sympathy lay in particular with the reduced families of Florence, and it was to bring help secretly to them–too proud to beg–that he called for volunteers. The society was known in the city as the Buonuomini (good men) of S. Martino, the little church close to Dante's house, behind the Badia: S. Martin being famous among saints for his impulsive yet wise generosity with his cloak.

The other and most famous prior of S. Marco was Savonarola. Girolamo Savonarola was born of noble family at Ferrara in 1452, and after a profound education, in which he concentrated chiefly upon religion and philosophy, he entered the Dominican order at the age of twenty-two. He first came to S. Marco at the age of thirty and preached there in Lent in 1482, but without attracting much notice. When, however, he returned to S. Marco seven years later it was to be instantly hailed both as a powerful preacher and reformer. His eloquent and burning declarations were hurled both at Florence and Rome: at the apathy and greed of the Church as a whole, and at the sinfulness and luxury of this city, while Lorenzo the Magnificent, who was then at the height of his influence, surrounded by accomplished and witty hedonists, and happiest when adding to his collection of pictures, jewels, and sculpture, in particular did the priest rebuke. Savonarola stood for the spiritual ideals and asceticism of the Baptist, Christ, and S. Paul; Lorenzo, in his eyes, made only for sensuality and decadence.

The two men, however, recognized each other's genius, and Lorenzo, with the tolerance which was as much a mark of the first three Medici rulers as its absence was notable in most of the later ones, rather encouraged Savonarola in his crusade than not. He visited him in the monastery and did not resent being kept waiting; and he went to hear him preach. In 1492 Lorenzo died, sending for Savonarola on his death-bed, which was watched by the two closest of his scholarly friends, Pico della Mirandola and Politian. The story of what happened has been variously told. According to the account of Politian, Lorenzo met his end with fortitude, and Savonarola prayed with the dying man and gave him his blessing; according to another account, Lorenzo was called upon by Savonarola to make three undertakings before he died, and, Lorenzo declining, Savonarola left him unabsolved. These promises were (1) to repent of all his sins, and in particular of the sack of Volterra, of the alleged theft of public dowry funds and of the implacable punishment of the Pazzi conspirators; (2) to restore all property of which he had become possessed by unjust means; and (3) to give back to Florence her liberty. But the probabilities are in favour of Politian's account being the true one, and the later story a political invention.

Lorenzo dead and Piero his son so incapable, Savonarola came to his own. He had long foreseen a revolution following on the death of Lorenzo, and in one of his most powerful sermons he had suggested that the "Flagellum Dei" to punish the wicked Florentines might be a foreign invader. When therefore in 1493 the French king Charles VIII arrived in Italy with his army, Savonarola was recognized not only as a teacher but as a prophet; and when the Medici had been again banished and Charles, having asked too much, had retreated from Florence, the Republic was remodelled with Savonarola virtually controlling its Great Council. For a year or two his power was supreme.

This was the period of the Piagnoni, or Weepers. The citizens adopted sober attire; a spirit as of England under the Puritans prevailed; and Savonarola's eloquence so far carried away not only the populace but many persons of genius that a bonfire was lighted in the middle of the Piazza della Signoria in which costly dresses, jewels, false hair and studies from the nude were destroyed.

Savonarola, meanwhile, was not only chastising and reforming Florence, but with fatal audacity was attacking with even less mincing of words the licentiousness of the Pope. As to the character of Lorenzo de' Medici there can be two opinions, and indeed the historians of Florence are widely divided in their estimates; but of Roderigo Borgia (Pope Alexander VI) there is but one, and Savonarola held it. Savonarola was excommunicated, but refused to obey the edict. Popes, however, although Florence had to a large extent put itself out of reach, have long arms, and gradually–taking advantage of the city's growing discontent with piety and tears and recurring unquiet, there being still a strong pro-Medici party, and building not a little on his knowledge of the Florentine love of change–the Pope gathered together sufficient supporters of his determination to crush this too outspoken critic and humiliate his fellow-citizens.

Events helped the pontiff. A pro-Medici conspiracy excited the populace; a second bonfire of vanities led to rioting, for the Florentines were beginning to tire of virtue; and the preaching of a Franciscan monk against Savonarola (and the gentle Fra Angelico has shown us, in the Accademia, how Franciscans and Dominicans could hate each other) brought matters to a head, for he challenged Savaronola to an ordeal by fire in the Loggia de' Lanzi, to test which of them spoke with the real voice of God. A Dominican volunteered to make the essay with a Franciscan. This ceremony, anticipated with the liveliest eagerness by the Florentines, was at the last moment forbidden, and Savonarola, who had to bear the responsibility of such a bitter disappointment to a pleasure-loving people, became an unpopular figure. Everything just then was against him, for Charles VIII, with whom he had an understanding and of whom the Pope was afraid, chose that moment to die.

The Pope drove home his advantage, and getting more power among individuals on the Council forced them to indict their firebrand. No means were spared, however base; forgery and false witness were as nothing. The summons arrived on April 8th, 1497, when Savonarola was at S. Marco. The monks, who adored him, refused to let him go, and for a whole day the convent was under siege. But might, of course, prevailed, and Savonarola was dragged from the church to the Palazzo Vecchio and prosecuted for the offence of claiming to have supernatural power and fomenting political disturbance. He was imprisoned in a tiny cell in the tower for many days, and under constant torture he no doubt uttered words which would never have passed his lips had he been in control of himself; but we may dismiss, as false, the evidence which makes them into confessions. Evidence there had to be, and evidence naturally was forthcoming; and sentence of death was passed.

In that cell, when not under torture, he managed to write meditations on the thirteenth psalm, "In Thee, O Lord, have I hoped," and a little work entitled "A Rule for Living a Christian Life". Before the last day he administered the Sacrament to his two companions, who were to die with him, with perfect composure, and the night preceding they spent together in prayer in the Great Hall which he had once dominated.

The execution was on May 23rd, 1498. A gallows was erected in the Piazza della Signoria on the spot now marked by the bronze tablet. Beneath the gallows was a bonfire. All those members of the Government who could endure the scene were present, either on the platform of the Palazzo Vecchio or in the Loggia de' Lanzi. The crowd filled the Piazza. The three monks went to their death unafraid. When his friar's gown was taken from him, Savonarola said: "Holy gown, thou wert granted to me by God's grace and I have ever kept thee unstained. Now I forsake thee not but am bereft of thee." (This very garment is in the glass case in Savonarola's cell at S. Marco.) The Bishop replied hastily: "I separate thee from the Church militant and triumphant". "Militant," replied Savonarola, "not triumphant, for that rests not with you." The monks were first hanged and then burned.

The larger picture of the execution which hangs in Savonarola's cell, although interesting and up to a point credible, is of course not right. The square must have been crowded: in fact we know it was. The picture has still other claims on the attention, for it shows the Judith and Holofernes as the only statue before the Palazzo Vecchio, standing where David now is; it shows the old ringhiera, the Marzocco (very inaccurately drawn), and the Loggia de' Lanzi empty of statuary. We have in the National Gallery a little portrait of Savonarola–No. 1301–with another representation of the execution on the back of it.

So far as I can understand Savonarola, his failure was due to two causes: firstly, his fatal blending of religion and politics, and secondly, the conviction which his temporary success with the susceptible Florentines bred in his heated mind that he was destined to carry all before him, totally failing to appreciate the Florentine character with all its swift and deadly changes and love of change. As I see it, Savonarola's special mission at that time was to be a wandering preacher, spreading the light and exciting his listeners to spiritual revival in this city and that, but never to be in a position of political power and never to become rooted. The peculiar tragedy of his career is that he left Florence no better than he found it: indeed, very likely worse; for in a reaction from a spiritual revival a lower depth can be reached than if there had been no revival at all; while the visit of the French army to Italy, for which Savonarola took such credit to himself, merely ended in disaster for Italy, disease for Europe, and the spreading of the very Renaissance spirit which he had toiled to destroy. But, when all is said as to his tragedy, personal and political, there remains this magnificent isolated figure, single-minded, austere and self-sacrificing, in an age of indulgence.

For most people "Romola" is the medium through which Savonarola is visualized; but there he is probably made too theatrical. Yet he must have had something of the theatre in him even to consent to the ordeal by fire. That he was an intense visionary is beyond doubt, but a very real man too we must believe when we read of the devotion of his monks to his person, and of his success for a while with the shrewd, worldly Great Council.

Savonarola had many staunch friends among the artists. We have seen Lorenzo di Credi and Fra Bartolommeo under his influence. After his death Fra Bartolommeo entered S. Marco (his cell was No. 34), and di Credi, who was noted for his clean living, entered S. Maria Nuova. Two of Luca della Robbia's nephews were also monks under Savonarola. We have seen Fra Bartolommeo's portrait of Savonarola in the Accademia, and there is another of him here. Cronaca, who built the Great Council's hall, survived Savonarola only ten years, and during that time all his stories were of him. Michelangelo, who was a young man when he heard him preach, read his sermons to the end of his long life. But upon Botticelli his influence was most powerful, for he turned that master's hand from such pagan allegories as the "Primavera" and the "Birth of Venus" wholly to religious subjects.

Savonarola had three adjoining cells. In the first is a monument to him, his portrait by Fra Bartolommeo and three frescoes by the same hand. In the next room is the glass case containing his robe, his hair shirt, and rosary; and here also are his desk and some books. In the bedroom is a crucifixion by Fra Angelico on linen. No one knowing Savonarola's story can remain here unmoved.

We find Fra Bartolommeo again with a pencil drawing of S. Antonio in that saint's cell. Here also is Antonino's death-mask. The terra-cotta bust of him in Cosimo's cell is the most like life, but there is an excellent and vivacious bronze in the right transept of S. Maria Novella.

Before passing downstairs again the library should be visited, that delightful assemblage of grey pillars and arches. Without its desks and cases it would be one of the most beautiful rooms in Florence. All the books have gone, save the illuminated music.

In the first cloisters, which are more liveable-in than the ordinary Florentine cloisters, having a great shady tree in the midst with a seat round it, and flowers, are the Fra Angelicos I have mentioned. The other painting is rather theatrical and poor. In the refectory is a large scene of the miracle of the Providenza, when S. Dominic and his companions, during a famine, were fed by two angels with bread; while at the back S. Antonio watches the crucified Christ. The artist is Sogliano.

In addition to Fra Angelico's great crucifixion fresco in the chapter house, is a single Christ crucified, with a monk mourning, by Antonio Pollaiuolo, very like the Fra Angelico in the cloisters; but the colour has left it, and what must have been some noble cypresses are now ghosts dimly visible. The frame is superb.

One other painting we must see–the "Last Supper" of Domenico Ghirlandaio. Florence has two "Last Suppers" by this artist–one at the Ognissanti and this. The two works are very similar and have much entertaining interest, but the debt which this owes to Castagno is very obvious: it is indeed Castagno sweetened. Although psychologically this picture is weak, or at any rate not strong, it is full of pleasant touches: the supper really is a supper, as it too often is not, with fruit and dishes and a generous number of flasks; the table-cloth would delight a good housekeeper; a cat sits close to Judas, his only companion; a peacock perches in a niche; there are flowers on the wall, and at the back of the charming loggia where the feast is held are luxuriant trees, and fruits, and flying birds. The monks at food in this small refectory had compensation for their silence in so engaging a scene. This room also contains a beautiful della Robbia "Deposition".

The little refectory, which is at the foot of the stairs leading to the cells, opens on the second cloisters, and these few visitors ever enter. But they are of deep interest to any one with a passion for the Florence of the great days, for it is here that the municipality preserves the most remarkable relics of buildings that have had to be destroyed. It is in fact the museum of the ancient city. Here, for example, is that famous figure of Abundance, in grey stone, which Donatello made for the old market, where the Piazza Vittorio Emmanuele now is, in the midst of which she poured forth her fruits from a cornucopia high on a column for all to see. Opposite is a magnificent doorway designed by Donatello for the Pazzi garden. Old windows, chimney-pieces, fragments of cornice, carved pillars, painted beams, coats of arms, are everywhere.

In cell No. 3 is a pretty little coloured relief of the Virgin adoring, which I covet, from a tabernacle in the old Piazza di Brunelleschi. Here too are relics of the guild houses of some of the smaller Arti, while perhaps the most humanly interesting thing of all is the great mournful bell of S. Marco in

Savonarola's time, known as La Piagnone.

In the church of S. Marco lie two of the learned men, friends of Lorenzo de' Medici, whose talk at the Medici table was one of the youthful Michelangelo's educative influences, what time he was studying in the Medici garden, close by: Angelo Poliziano (1454-1494), the poet and the tutor of the three Medici boys, and the marvellous Pico della Mirandola (1463-1494), the enchanted scholar. Pico was one of the most fascinating and comely figures of his time. He was born in 1463, the son of the Count of Mirandola, and took early to scholarship, spending his time among philosophies as other boys among games or S. Antonio at his devotions, but by no means neglecting polished life too, for we know him to have been handsome, accomplished, and a knight in the court of Venus. In 1486 he challenged the whole world to meet him in Rome and dispute publicly upon nine hundred theses; but so many of them seemed likely to be paradoxes against the true faith, too brilliantly defended, that the Pope forbade the contest. Pico dabbled in the black arts, wrote learnedly (in his room at the Badia of Fiesole) on the Mosaic law, was an amorous poet in Italian as well as a serious poet in Latin, and in everything he did was interesting and curious, steeped in Renaissance culture, and inspired by the wish to reconcile the past and the present and humanize Christ and the Fathers. He found time also to travel much, and he gave most of his fortune to establish a fund to provide penniless girls with marriage portions. He had enough imagination to be the close friend both of Lorenzo de' Medici and Savonarola. Savonarola clothed his dead body in Dominican robes and made him posthumously one of the order which for some time before his death he had desired to join. He died in 1494 at the early age of thirty-one, two years after Lorenzo.

Angelo Poliziano, known as Politian, was also a Renaissance scholar and also a friend of Lorenzo, and his companion, with Pico, at his death-bed; but although in precocity, brilliancy of gifts, and literary charm he may be classed with Pico, the comparison there ends, for he was a gross sensualist of mean exterior and capable of much pettiness. He was tutor to Lorenzo's sons until their mother interfered, holding that his views were far too loose, but while in that capacity he taught also Michelangelo and put him upon the designing of his relief of the battle of the Lapithae and Centaurs. At the time of Lorenzo and Giuliano's famous tournament in the Piazza of S. Croce, Poliziano wrote, as I have said, the descriptive allegorical poem which gave Botticelli ideas for his "Birth of Venus" and "Primavera". He lives chiefly by his Latin poems; but he did much to make the language of Tuscany a literary tongue. His elegy on the death of Lorenzo has real feeling in it and proves him to have esteemed that friend and patron. Like Pico, he survived Lorenzo only two years, and he also was buried in Dominican robes. Perhaps the finest feat of Poliziano's life was his action in slamming the sacristy doors in the face of Lorenzo's pursuers on that fatal day in the Duomo when Giuliano de' Medici was stabbed.

Ghirlandaio's fresco in S. Trinità of the granting of the charter to S. Francis gives portraits both of Poliziano and Lorenzo in the year 1485. Lorenzo stands in a little group of four in the right-hand corner, holding out his hand towards Poliziano, who, with Lorenzo's son Giuliano on his right and followed by two other boys, is advancing up the steps. Poliziano is seen again in a Ghirlandaio fresco at S. Maria Novella.

From S. Marco we are going to SS. Annunziata, but first let us just take a few steps down the Via Cavour, in order to pass the Casino Medici, since it is built on the site of the old Medici garden where Lorenzo de' Medici established Bertoldo, the sculptor, as head of a school of instruction, amid those beautiful antiques which we have seen in the Uffizi, and where the boy Michelangelo was a student.

A few steps farther on the left, towards the Fiesole heights, which we can see rising at the end of the street, we come, at No. 69, to a little doorway which leads to a little courtyard–the Chiostro dello Scalzo–decorated with frescoes by Andrea del Sarto and Franciabigio and containing the earliest work of both artists. The frescoes are in monochrome, which is very unusual, but their interest is not impaired thereby: one does not miss other colours. No. 7, the Baptism of Christ, is the first fresco these two associates ever did; and several years elapsed between that and the best that are here, such as the group representing Charity and the figure of Faith, for the work was long interrupted. The boys on the staircase in the fresco which shows S. John leaving his father's house are very much alive. This is by Franciabigio, as is also S. John meeting with Christ, a very charming scene. Andrea's best and latest is the Birth of the Baptist, which has the fine figure of Zacharias writing in it. But what he should be writing at that time and place one cannot imagine: more reasonably might he be called a physician preparing a prescription. On the wall is a terra-cotta bust of S. Antonio, making him much younger than is usual.

Andrea's suave brush we find all over Florence, both in fresco and picture, and this is an excellent place to say something of the man of whom English people have perhaps a more intimate impression than of any other of the old masters, by reason largely of Browning's poem and not a little by that beautiful portrait which for so long was erroneously considered to represent the painter himself, in our National Gallery. Andrea's life was not very happy. No painter had more honour in his own day, and none had a greater number of pupils, but these stopped with him only a short time, owing to the demeanour towards them of Andrea's wife, who developed into a flirt and shrew, dowered with a thousand jealousies. Andrea, the son of a tailor, was born in 1486 and apprenticed to a goldsmith. Showing, however, more drawing than designing ability, he was transferred to a painter named Barile and then passed to that curious man of genius who painted the fascinating picture "The Death of Procris" which hangs near Andrea's portrait in our National Gallery–Piero di Cosimo. Piero carried oddity to strange lengths. He lived alone in indescribable dirt, and lived wholly on hard-boiled eggs, which he cooked, with his glue, by the fifty, and ate as he felt inclined. He forbade all pruning of trees as an act of insubordination to Nature, and delighted in rain but cowered in terror from thunder and lightning. He peered curiously at clouds to find strange shapes in them, and in his pursuit of the grotesque examined the spittle of sick persons on the walls or ground, hoping for suggestions of monsters, combats of horses, or fantastic landscapes. But why this should have been thought madness in Cosimo when Leonardo in his directions to artists explicitly advises them to look hard at spotty walls for inspiration, I cannot say. He was also the first, to my knowledge, to don ear-caps in tedious society–as Herbert Spencer later used to do. He had many pupils, but latterly could not bear them in his presence and was therefore but an indifferent instructor. As a deviser of pageants he was more in demand than as a painter; but his brush was not idle. Both London and Paris have, I think, better examples of his genius than the Uffizi; but he is well represented at S. Spirito.

Piero sent Andrea to the Palazzo Vecchio to study the Leonardo and Michelangelo cartoons, and there he met Franciabigio, with whom he struck up one of his close friendships, and together they took a studio and began to paint for a living. Their first work together was the Baptism of Christ at which we are now looking. The next commission after the Scalzo was to decorate the courtyard of the Convent of the Servi, now known as the Church of the Annunciation; and moving into adjacent lodgings, Andrea met Jacopo Sansovino, the Venetian sculptor, whose portrait by Bassano is in the Uffizi, a capable all-round man who had studied in Rome and was in the way of helping the young Andrea at all points. It was then too that he met the agreeable and convivial Rustici, of whom I have said something in the chapter on the Baptistery, and quickly became something of a blood–for by this time, the second decade of the sixteenth century, the simplicity of the early artists had given place to dashing sophistication and the great period was nearly over. For this change the brilliant complex inquiring mind of Leonardo da Vinci was largely responsible, together with the encouragement and example of Lorenzo de' Medici and such of his cultured sceptical friends as Alberti, Pico della Mirandola, and Poliziano. But that is a subject too large for this book. Enough that a worldly splendour and vivacity had come into artistic life and Andrea was an impressionable young man in the midst of it. It does not seem to have affected the power and dexterity of his hand, but it made him a religious court-painter instead of a religious painter. His sweetness and an underlying note of pathos give his work a peculiar and genuine character; but he is just not of the greatest. Not so great really as Luca Signorelli, for example, whom few visitors to the galleries rush at with gurgling cries of rapture as they rush at Andrea.

When Andrea was twenty-six he married. The lady was the widow of a hatter. Andrea had long loved her, but the hatter clung outrageously to life. In 1513, however, she was free, and, giving her hand to the painter, his freedom passed for ever. Vasari being among Andrea's pupils may be trusted here, and Vasari gives her a bad character, which Browning completes. Andrea painted her often, notably in the fresco of the "Nativity of the Virgin," to which we shall soon come at the Annunziata: a fine statuesque woman by no means unwilling to have the most popular artist in Florence as her slave.

Of the rest of Andrea's life I need say little. He grew steadily in favour and was always busy; he met Michelangelo and admired him, and Michelangelo warned Raphael in Rome of a little fellow in Florence who would "make him sweat". Browning, in his monologue, makes this remark of Michelangelo's, and the comparison between Andrea and Raphael that follows, the kernel of the poem.

Like Leonardo and Rustici, Andrea accepted, in 1518, an invitation from Francis I to visit Paris and once there began to paint for that royal patron. But although his wife did not love him, she wanted him back, and in the midst of his success he returned, taking with him a large sum of money from Francis with which to buy for the king works of art in Italy. That money he misapplied to his own extravagant ends, and although Francis took no punitive steps, the event cannot have improved either Andrea's position or his peace of mind; while it caused Francis to vow that he had done with Florentines. Andrea died in 1531, of fever, nursed by no one, for his wife, fearing it might be the dreaded plague, kept away.

CHAPTER XIX

THE SS. Annunziata and the Spedale degli Innocenti

Andrea del Sarto again–Franciabigio outraged–Alessio Baldovinetti–Piero de' Medici's church–An Easter Sunday congregation–Andrea's "Madonna del Sacco"–"The Statue and the Bust"–Henri IV–The Spedale degli Innocenti–Andrea della Robbia–Domenico Ghirlandaio–Cosimo I and the Etruscans–Bronzes and tapestries–Perugino's triptych–S. Mary Magdalene de' Pazzi–"Very sacred human dust".

From S. Marco it is an easy step, along the Via Sapienza, to the Piazza dell' Annunziata, where one finds the church of that name, the Palazzo Riccardi-Mannelli, and opposite it, gay with the famous della Robbia reliefs of swaddled children, the Spedale degli Innocenti.

First the church, which is notable for possessing in its courtyard Andrea del Sarto's finest frescoes. This series, of which he was the chief painter, with his friend Franciabigio again as his principal ally, depict scenes in the life of the Virgin and S. Filippo. The scene of the Birth of the Virgin has been called the triumph of fresco painting, and certainly it is very gay and life-like in that medium. The whole picture very charming and easy, with the pleasantest colouring imaginable and pretty details, such as the washing of the baby and the boy warming his hands, while of the two women in the foreground, that on the left, facing the spectator, is a portrait of Andrea's wife, Lucrezia. In the Arrival of the Magi we find Andrea himself, the figure second from the right-hand side, pointing; while next to him, on the left, is his friend Jacopo Sansovino. The "Dead Man Restored to Life by S. Filippo" is Andrea's next best. Franciabigio did the scene of the Marriage of the Virgin, which contains another of his well-drawn boys on the steps. The injury to this fresco–the disfigurement of Mary's face–was the work of the painter himself, in a rage that the monks should have inspected it before it was ready. Vasari is interesting on this work. He draws attention to it as illustrating "Joseph's great faith in taking her, his face expressing as much fear as joy". He also says that the blow which the man is giving Joseph was part of the marriage ceremony at that time in Florence.

Franciabigio, in spite of his action in the matter of this fresco, seems to have been a very sweet-natured man, who painted rather to be able to provide for his poor relations than from any stronger inner impulse, and when he saw some works by Raphael gave up altogether, as Verrocchio gave up after Leonardo matured. Franciabigio was a few years older than Andrea, but died at the same age. Possibly it was through watching his friend's domestic troubles that he remained single, remarking that he who takes a wife endures strife. His most charming work is that "Madonna of the Well" in the Uffizi, which is reproduced in this volume. Franciabigio's master was Mariotto Albertinelli, who had learned from Cosimo Rosselli, the teacher of Piero di Cosimo, Andrea's master–another illustration of the interdependence of Florentine artists.

One of the most attractive works in the courtyard must once have been the "Adoration of the Shepherds" by Alessio Baldovinetti, at the left of the entrance to the church. It is badly damaged and the colour has gone, but one can see that the valley landscape, when it was painted, was a dream of gaiety and happiness.

The particular treasure of the church is the extremely ornate chapel of the Virgin, containing a picture of the Virgin displayed once a year on the Feast of the Annunciation, March 25th, in the painting of which the Virgin herself took part, descending from heaven for that purpose. The artist thus divinely assisted was Pietro Cavallini, a pupil of Giotto. The silver shrine for the picture was designed by Michelozzo and was a beautiful thing before the canopy and all the distressing accessories were added. It was made at the order of Piero de' Medici, who was as fond of this church as his father Cosimo was of S. Lorenzo. Michelozzo only designed it; the sculpture was done by Pagno di Lapo Portigiani, whose Madonna is over the tomb of Pope John by Donatello and Michelozzo in the Baptistery.

Among the altar-pieces are two by Perugino; but of Florentine altar-pieces one can say little or nothing in a book of reasonable dimensions. There are so many and they are for the most part so difficult to see. Now and then one arrests the eye and holds it; but for the most part they go unstudied. The rotunda of the choir is interesting, for here we meet again Alberti, who completed it from designs by Michelozzo. It does not seem to fit the church from within, and even less so from without, but it is a fine structure. The seventeenth-century painting of the dome is almost impressive.

But one can forget and forgive all the church's gaudiness and floridity when the choir is in good voice and the strings play Palestrina as they did last Easter Sunday. The Annunziata is famous for its music, and on the great occasions people crowd there as nowhere else. At High Mass the singing was fine but the instrumental music finer. One is accustomed to seeing vicarious worship in Italy; but never was there so vicarious a congregation as ours, and indeed if it had not been for the sight of the busy celibates at the altar one would not have known that one was worshipping at all. The culmination of detachment came when a family of Siamese or Burmese children, in native dress, entered. A positive hum went round, and not an eye but was fixed on the little Orientals. When, however, the organ was for a while superseded and the violas and violins quivered under the plangent melody of Palestrina, our roving attention was fixed and held.

I am not sure that the Andrea in the cloisters is not the best of all his work. It is very simple and wholly beautiful, and in spite of years of ravage the colouring is still wonderful, perhaps indeed better for the hand of Time. It is called the "Madonna del Sacco" (grain sack), and fills the lunette over the door leading from the church. The Madonna–Andrea's favourite type, with the eyes set widely in the flat brow over the little trustful nose–has her Son, older than usual, sprawling on her knee. Her robes are ample and rich; a cloak of green is over her pretty head. By her sits S. Joseph, on the sack, reading with very long sight. That is all; but one does not forget it.

For the rest the cloisters are a huddle of memorial slabs and indifferent frescoes. In the middle is a well with nice iron work. No grass at all. The second cloisters, into which it is not easy to get, have a gaunt John the Baptist in terra-cotta by Michelozzo.

On leaving the church, our natural destination is the Spedale, on the left, but one should pause a moment in the doorway of the courtyard (if the beggars who are always there do not make it too difficult) to look down the Via de' Servi running straight away to the cathedral, which, with its great red warm dome, closes the street. The statue in the middle of the piazza is that of the Grand Duke Ferdinand by Giovanni da Bologna, cast from metal taken from the Italians' ancient enemies the Turks, while the fountains are by Tacca, Giovanni's pupil, who made the bronze boar at the Mercato Nuovo. "The Synthetical Guide Book," from which I have already quoted, warns its readers not to overlook "the puzzling bees" at the back of Ferdinand's statue. "Try to count them," it adds. (I accepted the challenge and found one hundred and one.) The bees have reference to Ferdinand's emblem–a swarm of these insects, with the words "Majestate tantum". The statue, by the way, is interesting for two other reasons than its subject. First, it is that to which Browning's poem, "The Statue and the Bust," refers, and which, according to the poet, was set here at Ferdinand's command to gaze adoringly for ever at the della Robbia bust of the lady whom he loved in vain. But the bust no longer is visible, if ever it was. John of Douay (as Gian Bologna was also called)–

John of Douay shall effect my plan, Set me on horseback here aloft, Alive, as the crafty sculptor can,

In the very square I have crossed so oft: That men may admire, when future suns Shall touch the eyes to a purpose soft,

While the mouth and the brow stay brave in bronze– Admire and say, "when he was alive How he would take his pleasure once!"

The other point of interest is that when Maria de' Medici, Ferdinand's niece, wished to erect a statue of Henri IV (her late husband) at the Pont Neuf in Paris she asked to borrow Gian Bologna. But the sculptor was too old to go and therefore only a bronze cast of this same horse was offered. In the end Tacca completed both statues, and Henri IV was set up in 1614 (after having fallen overboard on the voyage from Leghorn to Havre). The present statue at the Pont Neuf is, however, a modern substitute.

The façade of the Spedale degli Innocenti, or children's hospital, when first seen by the visitor evokes perhaps the quickest and happiest cry of recognition in all Florence by reason of its row of della Robbia babies, each in its blue circle, reproductions of which have gone all over the world. These are thought to be by Andrea, Luca's nephew, and were added long after the building was completed. Luca probably helped him. The hospital was begun by Brunelleschi at the cost of old Giovanni de' Medici, Cosimo's father, but the Guild of the Silk Weavers, for whom Luca made the exquisite coat of arms on Or San Michele, took it over and finished it. Andrea not only modelled the babies outside but the beautiful Annunciation (of which I give a reproduction in this volume) in the court: one of his best works. The photograph will show how full of pretty thoughts it is, but in colour it is more charming still and the green of the lily stalks is not the least delightful circumstance. Not only among works of sculpture but among Annunciations this relief holds a very high place. Few of the artists devised a scene in which the great news was brought more engagingly, in sweeter surroundings, or received more simply.

The door of the chapel close by leads to another work of art equally adapted to its situation–Ghirlandaio's Adoration of the Magi: one of the perfect pictures for children. We have seen Ghirlandaio's Adoration of the Shepherds at the Accademia: this is its own brother. It has the sweetest, mildest little Mother, and in addition to the elderly Magi two tiny little saintlings adore too. In the distance is an enchanted landscape about a fairy estuary.

This hospital is a very busy one, and the authorities are glad to show it to visitors who really take an interest in such work. Rich Italians carry on a fine rivalry in generosity to such institutions. Bologna, for instance, could probably give lessons in thoughtful charity to the whole world.

The building opposite the hospital has a loggia which is notable for a series of four arches, like those of the Mercato Nuovo, and in summer for the flowers that hang down from the little balconies. A pretty building. Before turning to the right under the last of the arches of the hospital loggia, which opens on the Via della Colonna and from the piazza always frames such a charming picture of houses and mountains, it is well, with so much of Andrea del Sarto's work warm in one's memory, to take a few steps up the Via Gino Capponi (which also always frames an Apennine vista under its arch) to No. 24, and see Andrea's house, on the right, marked with a tablet.

In the Via della Colonna we find, at No. 26 on the left, the Palazzo Crocetta, which is now a Museum of Antiquities, and for its Etruscan exhibits is of the greatest historical value and interest to visitors to Tuscany, such as ourselves. For here you may see what civilization was like centuries before Christ and Rome. The beginnings of the Etruscan people are indistinct, but about 1000 B.C. has been agreed to as the dawn of their era. Etruria comprised Tuscany, Perugia, and Rome itself. Florence has no remains, but Fiesole was a fortified Etruscan town, and many traces of its original builders may be seen there, together with Etruscan relics in the little museum. For the best reconstructions of an Etruscan city one must go to Volterra, where so many of the treasures in the present building were found.

The Etruscans in their heyday were the most powerful people in the world, but after the fifth century their supremacy gradually disappeared, the Gauls on the one side and the Romans on the other wearing them down. All our knowledge of them comes through the spade. Excavations at Volterra and elsewhere have revealed some thousands of inscriptions which have been in part deciphered; but nothing has thrown so much light on this accomplished people as their habit of providing the ashes of their dead with everything likely to be needed for the next world, whose requirements fortunately so exactly tallied with those of this that a complete system of domestic civilization can be deduced. In arts and sciences they were most enviably advanced, as a visit to the British Museum will show in a moment. But it is to this Florentine Museum of Antiquities that all students of Etruria must go. The garden contains a number of the tombs themselves, rebuilt and refurnished exactly as they were found; while on the ground floor is the amazing collection of articles which the tombs yielded. The grave has preserved them for us, not quite so perfectly as the volcanic dust of Vesuvius preserved the domestic appliances of Pompeii, but very nearly so. Jewels, vessels, weapons, ornaments–many of them of a beauty never since reproduced–are to be seen in profusion, now gathered together for study only a short distance from the districts in which centuries ago they were made and used for actual life.

Upstairs we find relics of an older civilization still, the Egyptian, and a few rooms of works of art, all found in Etruscan soil, the property of the Pierpont Morgans and George Saltings of that ancient day, who had collected them exactly as we do now. Certain of the statues are world-famous. Here, for example, in Sala IX, is the bronze Minerva which was found near Arezzo in 1554 by Cosimo's workmen. Here is the Chimæra, also from Arezzo in 1554, which Cellini restored for Cosimo and tells us about in his Autobiography. Here is the superb Orator from Lake Trasimene, another of Cosimo's discoveries.

In Sala X look at the bronze situla in an isolated glass case, of such a peacock blue as only centuries could give it. Upstairs in Sala XVI are many more Greek and Roman bronzes, among which I noticed a faun with two pipes as being especially good; while the little room leading from it has some fine life-size heads, including a noble one of a horse, and the famous Idolino on its elaborate pedestal–a full-length Greek bronze from the earth of Pesaro, where it was found in 1530.

The top floor is given to tapestries and embroideries. The collection is vast and comprises much foreign work; but Cosimo I introducing tapestry weaving into Florence, many of the examples come from the city's looms. The finest, or at any rate most interesting, series is that depicting the court of France under Catherine de' Medici, with portraits: very sumptuous and gay examples of Flemish work.

The trouble at Florence is that one wants the days to be ten times as long in order that one may see its wonderful possessions properly. Here is this dry-looking archaeological museum, with antipathetic custodians at the door who refuse to get change for twenty-lira pieces: nothing could be more unpromising than they or their building; and yet you find yourself instantly among countless vestiges of a past people who had risen to power and crumbled again before Christ was born–but at a time when man was so vastly more sensitive to beauty than he now is that every appliance for daily life was the work of an artist. Well, a collection like this demands days and days of patient examination, and one has only a few hours. Were I Joshua–had I his curious gift–it is to Florence I would straightway fare. The sun should stand still there: no rock more motionless.

Continuing along the Via della Colonna, we come, on the right, at No. 8, to the convent of S. Maria Maddalena de' Pazzi, which is now a barracks but keeps sacred one room in which Perugino painted a crucifixion, his masterpiece in fresco. The work is in three panels, of which that on the left, representing the Virgin and S. Bernard, is the most beautiful. Indeed, there is no more beautiful light in any picture we shall see, and the Virgin's melancholy face is inexpressibly sweet. Perugino is best represented at the Accademia, and there are works of his at the Uffizi and Pitti and in various Florentine churches; but here he is at his best. Vasari tells us that he made much money and was very fond of it; also that he liked his young wife to wear light head-dresses both out of doors and in the house, and often dressed her himself. His master was Verrocchio and his best pupil Raphael.

S. Mary Magdalene de' Pazzi, a member of the same family that plotted against the Medici and owned the sacred flints, was born in 1566, and, says Miss Dunbar, [8] "showed extraordinary piety from a very tender age". When only a child herself she used to teach small children, and she daily carried lunch to the prisoners. Her real name was Catherine, but becoming a nun she called herself Mary Magdalene. In an illness in which she was given up for dead, she lay on her bed for forty days, during which she saw continual visions, and then recovered. Like S. Catherine of Bologna she embroidered well and painted miraculously, and she once healed a leprosy by licking it. She died in 1607.

The old English Cemetery, as it is usually called–the Protestant Cemetery, as it should be called–is an oval garden of death in the Piazza Donatello, at the end of the Via di Pinti and the Via Alfieri, rising up from the boulevard that surrounds the northern half of Florence. (The new Protestant Cemetery is outside the city on the road to the Certosa.) I noticed, as I walked beneath the cypresses, the grave of Arthur Hugh Clough, the poet of "Dipsychus," who died here in Florence on November 13th, 1861; of Walter Savage Landor, that old lion (born January 30th, 1775; died September 17th, 1864), of whom I shall say much more in a later chapter; of his son Arnold, who was born in 1818 and died in 1871; and of Mrs. Holman Hunt, who died in 1866. But the most famous grave is that of Elizabeth Barrett Browning, who lies beneath a massive tomb that bears only the initials E.B.B. and the date 1861. "Italy," wrote James Thomson, the poet of "The City of Dreadful Night," on hearing of Mrs. Browning's death,

"Italy, you hold in trust Very sacred human dust."

CHAPTER XX

THE Cascine and the Arno

Florence's Bois de Boulogne–Shelley–The races–The game of Pallone–SS. Ognissanti–Botticelli and Ghirlandaio–Amerigo Vespucci–The Platonic Academy's garden–Alberti's Palazzo Rucellai–Melancholy decay–Two smiling boys–The Corsini palace–The Trinità bridge–The Borgo San Jacopo from the back–Home fishing–SS. Apostoli–A sensitive river–The Ponte Vecchio–The goldsmiths–S. Stefano.

The Cascine is the "Bois" of Florence; but it does not compare with the Parisian expanse either in size or attraction. Here the wealthy Florentines drive, the middle classes saunter and ride bicycles, the poor enjoy picnics, and the English take country walks. The further one goes the better it is, and the better also the river, which at the very end of the woods becomes such a stream as the pleinairistes love, with pollarded trees on either side. Among the trees of one of these woods nearly a hundred years ago, a walking Englishman named Percy Bysshe Shelley wrote his "Ode to the West Wind".

The Cascine is a Bois also in having a race-course in it–a small course with everything about it on a little scale, grandstand, betting boxes, and all. And why not?–for after all Florence is quite small in size, however remarkable in character. Here funny little race-meetings are held, beginning on Easter Monday and continuing at intervals until the weather gets too hot. The Florentines pour out in their hundreds and lie about in the long grass among the wild flowers, and in their fives and tens back their fancies. The system is the pari-mutuel, and here one seems to be more at its mercy even than in France. The odds keep distressingly low; but no one seems to be either elated or depressed, whatever happens. To be at the races is the thing–to walk about and watch the people and enjoy the air. It is the most orderly frugal scene, and the baleful and mysterious power of the racehorse to poison life and landscape, as in England, does not exist here.

To the Cascine also in the spring and autumn several hundred Florentine men come every afternoon to see the game of pallone and risk a few lire on their favourite players. Mr. Ruskin, whose "Mornings in Florence" is still the textbook of the devout, is severe enough upon those visitors who even find it in their hearts to shop and gossip in the city of Giotto. What then would he have said of one who has spent not a few afternoon hours, between five and six, in watching the game of pallone? I would not call pallone a good game. Compared with tennis, it is nothing; compared with lawn tennis, it is poor; compared with football, it is anaemic; yet in an Italian city, after the galleries have closed, on a warm afternoon, it will do, and it will more than do as affording an opportunity of seeing muscular Italian athletes in the pink of condition. The game is played by six, three each side: a battitore, who smites the ball, which is served to him very much as in rounders; the spalla, who plays back; and the terzino, who plays forward. The court is sixty or more yards long, on one side being a very high wall and on the other and at each end netting. The implements are the ball, which is hollow and of leather, about half the size of a football, and a cylinder studded with spikes, rather like a huge fir-cone or pine-apple, which is placed over the wrist and forearm to hit the ball with; and the game is much as in tennis, only there is no central net: merely a line. Each man's ambition, however, is less to defeat the returning power of the foe than to paralyse it by hitting the ball out of reach. It is as though a batsman were out if he failed to hit three wides.

A good battitore, for instance, can smite the ball right down the sixty yards into the net, above the head of the opposing spalla who stands awaiting it at the far end. Such a stroke is to the English mind a blot, and it is no uncommon thing, after each side has had a good rally, to see the battitore put every ball into the net in this way and so win the game without his opponents having one return; which is the very negation of sport. Each innings lasts until one side has gained eight points, the points going to whichever player makes the successful stroke. This means that the betting–and of course there is betting–is upon individuals and not upon sides.

The pari-mutuel system is that which is adopted at both the pallone courts in Florence (there is another at the Piazza Beccaria), and the unit is two lire. Bets are invited on the winner and the second, and place-money is paid on both. No wonder then that as the game draws to a close the excitement becomes intense; while during its progress feeling runs high too. For how can a young Florentine who has his money on, say, Gabri the battitore, withhold criticism when Gabri's arm fails and the ball drops comfortably for the terzino Ugo to smash it into Gabri's net? Such a lapse should not pass unnoticed; nor does it.

From the Cascine we may either return to Florence along the banks of the river, or cross the river by the vile iron Ponte Sospeso and enter the city again, on the Pitti side, by the imposing Porta S. Frediano. Supposing that we return by the Lungarno Amerigo Vespucci there is little to notice, beyond costly modern houses of a Portland Place type and the inevitable Garibaldi statue, until, just past the oblique pescaja (or weir), we see across the Piazza Manin the church of All Saints–S. Salvadore d'Ognissanti, which must be visited since it is the burial-place of Botticelli and Amerigo Vespucci, the chapel of the Vespucci family being painted by Ghirlandaio; and since here too lies Botticelli's beautiful Simonetta, who so untimely died. According to Vasari the frescoes of S. Jerome by Ghirlandaio and S. Augustine by Botticelli were done in competition. They were painted, as it happens, elsewhere, but moved here without injury. I think the S. Jerome is the more satisfying, a benevolent old scientific author–a Lord Avebury of the canon–with his implements about him on a tapestry tablecloth, a brass candlestick, his cardinal's hat, and a pair of tortoise-shell eyeglasses handy. S. Augustine is also scientific; astronomical books and instruments surround him too. His tablecloth is linen.

Amerigo Vespucci, whose statue we saw in the Uffizi portico colonnade, was a Florentine by birth who settled in Spain and took to exploration. His discoveries were important, but America is not really among them, for Columbus, whom he knew and supported financially, got there first. By a mistake in the date in his account of his travels, Vespucci's name came to be given to the new continent, and it was then too late to alter it. He became a naturalized Spaniard and died in 1512. Columbus indeed suffers in Florence; for had it not been for Vespucci, America would no doubt be called Columbia; while Brunelleschi anticipated him in the egg trick.

The church is very proud of possessing the robe of S. Francis, which is displayed once a year on October 4th. In the refectory is a "Last Supper" by Ghirlandaio, not quite so good as that which we saw at S. Marco, but very similar, and, like that, deriving from Castagno's at the Cenacolo di Sant' Apollonia. The predestined Judas is once more on the wrong side of the table.

Returning to the river bank again, we are at once among the hotels and pensions, which continue cheek by jowl right away to the Ponte Vecchio and beyond. In the Piazza Goldoni, where the Ponte Carraia springs off, several streets meet, best of them and busiest of them being that Via della Vigna Nuova which one should miss few opportunities of walking along, for here is the palazzo–at No. 20–which Leon Battista Alberti designed for the Rucellai. The Rucellai family's present palace, I may say here, is in the Via della Scala, and by good fortune I found at the door sunning himself a complacent major-domo who, the house being empty of its august owners, allowed me to walk through into the famous garden–the Orti Oricellari–where the Platonic Academy met for a while in Bernardo Rucellai's day. A monument inscribed with their names has been erected among the evergreens. Afterwards the garden was given by Francis I to his beloved Bianca Capella. Its natural beauties are impaired by a gigantic statue of Polyphemus, bigger than any other statue in Florence.

The new Rucellai palace does not compare with the old, which is, I think, the most beautiful of all the private houses of the great day, and is more easily seen too, for there is a little piazza in front of it. The palace, with its lovely design and its pilastered windows, is now a rookery, while various industries thrive beneath it. Part of the right side has been knocked away; but even still the proportions are noble. This is a bad quarter for vandalism; for in the piazza opposite is a most exquisite little loggia, built in 1468, the three lovely arches of which have been filled in and now form the windows of an English establishment known as "The Artistic White House". An absurd name, for if it were really artistic it would open up the arches again.

The Rucellai chapel, behind the palace, is in the Via della Spada, and the key must be asked for in the palace stables. It is in a shocking state, and quite in keeping with the traditions of the neighbourhood, while the old church of S. Pancrazio, its neighbour, is now a Government tobacco factory. The Rucellai chapel contains a model of the Holy Sepulchre, at Jerusalem, in marble and intarsia, by the great Alberti–one of the most jewel-like little buildings imaginable. Within it are the faint vestiges of a fresco which the stable-boy calls a Botticelli, and indeed the hands and faces of the angels, such as one can see of them with a farthing dip, do not render the suggestion impossible. On the altar is a terra-cotta Christ which he calls a Donatello, and again he may be right; but fury at a condition of things that can permit such a beautiful place to be so desecrated renders it impossible to be properly appreciative.

Since we are here, instead of returning direct to the river let us go a few yards along this Via della Spada to the left, cross the Via de' Fossi, and so come to the busy Via di Pallazzuolo, on the left of which, past the piazza of S. Paolino, is the little church of S. Francesco de' Vanchetoni. This church is usually locked, but the key is next door, on the right, and it has to be obtained because over the right sacristy door is a boy's head by Rossellino, and over the left a boy's head by Desiderio da Settignano, and each is joyful and perfect.

The Via de' Fossi will bring us again to the Piazza Goldoni and the Arno, and a few yards farther along there is a palace to be seen, the Corsini, the only palazzo still inhabited by its family to which strangers are admitted–the long low white façade with statues on the top and a large courtyard, on the Lungarno Corsini, just after the Piazza Goldoni. It is not very interesting and belongs to the wrong period, the seventeenth century. It is open on fixed days, and free save that one manservant receives the visitor and another conducts him from room to room. There are many pictures, but few of outstanding merit, and the authorship of some of these has been challenged. Thus, the cartoon of Julius II, which is called a Raphael and seems to be the sketch for one of the well-known portraits at the Pitti, Uffizi, or our National Gallery, is held to be not by Raphael at all. Among the pleasantest pictures are a Lippo Lippi Madonna and Child, a Filippino Lippi Madonna and Child with Angels, and a similar group by Botticelli; but one has a feeling that Carlo Dolci and Guido Reni are the true heroes of the house. Guido Reni's Lucrezia Romana, with a dagger which she has already thrust two inches into her bosom, as though it were cheese, is one of the most foolish pictures I ever saw. The Corsini family having given the world a pope, a case of papal vestments is here. It was this Pope when Cardinal Corsini who said to Dr. Johnson's friend, Mrs. Piozzi, meeting him in Florence in 1785, "Well, Madam, you never saw one of us red-legged partridges before, I believe".

There may be more beautiful bridges in the world than the Trinità, but I have seen none. Its curve is so gentle and soft, and its three arches so light and graceful, that I wonder that whenever new bridges are necessary the authorities do not insist upon the Trinità being copied. The Ponte Vecchio, of course, has a separate interest of its own, and stands apart, like the Rialto. It is a bridge by chance, one might almost say. But the Trinità is a bridge in intent and supreme at that, the most perfect union of two river banks imaginable. It shows to what depths modern Florence can fall–how little she esteems her past–that the iron bridge by the Cascine should ever have been built.

The various yellows of Florence–the prevailing colours–are spread out nowhere so favourably as on the Pitti side of the river between the Trinità and the Ponte Vecchio on the backs of the houses of the Borgo San Jacopo, and just so must this row have looked for four hundred years. Certain of the occupants of these tenements, even on the upper floors, have fishing nets, on pulleys, which they let down at intervals during the day for the minute fish which seem to be as precious to Italian fishermen as sparrows and wrens to Italian gunners.

The great palace at the Trinità end of this stretch of yellow buildings–the Frescobaldi–must have been very striking when the loggia was open: the three rows of double arches that are now walled in. From this point, as well as from similar points on the other side of the Ponte Vecchio, one realizes the mischief done by Cosimo I's secret passage across it; for not only does the passage impose a straight line on a bridge that was never intended to have one, but it cuts Florence in two. If it were not for its large central arches one would, from the other bridges or the embankment, see nothing whatever of the further side of the city; but as it is, through these arches one has heavenly vignettes.

We leave the river again for a few minutes about fifty yards along the Lungarno Acciaioli beyond the Trinità and turn up a narrow passage to see the little church of SS. Apostoli, where there is a delightful gay ciborium, all bright colours and happiness, attributed to Andrea della Robbia, with pretty cherubs and pretty angels, and a benignant Christ and flowers and fruit which cannot but chase away gloom and dubiety. Here also is a fine tomb by the sculptor of the elaborate chimney-piece which we saw in the Bargello,

Benedetto da Rovezzano, who also designed the church's very beautiful door. Whether or not it is true that SS. Apostoli was built by Charlemagne, it is certainly very old and architecturally of great interest. Vasari says that Brunelleschi acquired from it his inspiration for S. Lorenzo and S. Spirito. To many Florentines its principal importance is its custody of the Pazzi flints for the igniting of the sacred fire which in turn ignites the famous Carro.

Returning again to the embankment, we are quickly at the Ponte Vecchio, where it is pleasant at all times to loiter and observe both the river and the people; while from its central arches one sees the mountains. From no point are the hill of S. Miniato and its stately cypresses more beautiful; but one cannot see the church itself–only the church of S. Niccolò below it, and of course the bronze "David". In dry weather the Arno is green; in rainy weather yellow. It is so sensitive that one can almost see it respond to the most distant shower; but directly the rain falls and it is fed by a thousand Apennine torrents it foams past this bridge in fury. The Ponte Vecchio was the work, upon a Roman foundation, of Taddeo Gaddi, Giotto's godson, in the middle of the fourteenth century, but the shops are, of course, more recent. The passage between the Pitti and Uffizi was added in 1564. Gaddi, who was a fresco painter first and architect afterwards, was employed because Giotto was absent in Milan, Giotto being the first thought of every one in difficulties at that time. The need, however, was pressing, for a flood in 1333 had destroyed a large part of the Roman bridge. Gaddi builded so well that when, two hundred and more years later, another flood severely damaged three other bridges, the Ponte Vecchio was unharmed. None the less it is not Gaddi's bust but Cellini's that has the post of honour in the centre; but this is, of course, because Cellini was a goldsmith, and it is to goldsmiths that the shops belong. Once it was the butchers' quarter!

I never cross the Ponte Vecchio and see these artificers in their blouses through the windows, without wondering if in any of their boy assistants is the Michelangelo, or Orcagna, or Ghirlandaio, or even Cellini, of the future, since all of those, and countless others of the Renaissance masters, began in precisely this way.

The odd thing is that one is on the Ponte Vecchio, from either end, before one knows it to be a bridge at all. A street of sudden steepness is what it seems to be. Not the least charming thing upon it is the masses of groundsel which have established themselves on the pent roof over the goldsmiths' shops. Every visitor to Florence must have longed to occupy one of these little bridge houses; but I am not aware that any has done so.

One of the oldest streets in Florence must be the Via Girolami, from the Ponte Vecchio to the Uffizi, under an arch. A turning to the left brings one to the Piazza S. Stefano, where the barn-like church of S. Stefano is entered; and close by is the Torre de' Girolami, where S. Zenobius lived. S. Stefano, although it is now so easily overlooked, was of importance in its day, and it was here that Niccolò da Uzzano, the leader of the nobles, held a meeting to devise means of checking the growing power of the people early in the fifteenth century and was thwarted by old Giovanni de' Medici. From that thwarting proceeded the power of the Medici family and the gloriously endowed Florence that we travel to see.

CHAPTER XXI

. Maria Novella

S
The great churches of Florence–A Dominican cathedral–The "Decameron" begins–Domenico Ghirlandaio–Alessio Baldovinetti–The Louvre–The S. Maria Novella frescoes–Giovanni and Lorenzo Tornabuoni–Ruskin implacable–Cimabue's Madonna–Filippino Lippi–Orcagna's "Last Judgment"–The Cloisters of Florence–The Spanish Chapel–S. Dominic triumphant–Giotto at his sweetest–The "Wanderer's" doom–The Piazza, as an arena.

S. Maria Novella is usually bracketed with S. Croce as the most interesting Florentine church after the Duomo, but S. Lorenzo has of course to be reckoned with very seriously. I think that for interest I should place S. Maria Novella fifth, including also the Baptistery before it, but architecturally second. Its interior is second in beauty only to S. Croce. S. Croce is its immediate religious rival, for it was because the Dominicans had S. Maria Novella, begun in 1278, that several years later the Franciscans determined to have an equally important church and built S. Croce. The S. Maria Novella architects were brothers of the order, but Talenti, whom we saw at work both on Giotto's tower and on San Michele, built the campanile, and Leon Battista Alberti the marble façade, many years later. The richest patrons of S.

Maria Novella–corresponding to the Medici at S. Lorenzo and the Bardi at S. Croce–were the Rucellai, whose palace, designed also by the wonderful versatile Alberti, we have seen.

The interior of S. Maria Novella is very fine and spacious, and it gathers and preserves an exquisite light at all times of the day. Nowhere in Florence is there a finer aisle, with the roof springing so nobly and masterfully from the eight columns on either side. The whole effect, like that of S. Croce, is rather northern, the result of the yellow and brown hues; but whereas S. Croce has a crushing flat roof, this one is all soaring gladness.

The finest view of the interior is from the altar steps looking back to the beautiful circular window over the entrance, a mass of happy colour. In the afternoon the little plain circular windows high up in the aisle shoot shafts of golden light upon the yellow walls. The high altar of inlaid marble is, I think, too bright and too large. The church is more impressive on Good Friday, when over this altar is built a Calvary with the crucifix on the summit and life-size mourners at its foot; while a choir and string orchestra make superbly mournful music.

I like to think that it was within the older S. Maria Novella that those seven mirthful young ladies of Florence remained one morning in 1348, after Mass, to discuss plans of escape from the city during the plague. As here they chatted and plotted, there entered the church three young men; and what simpler than to engage them as companions in their retreat, especially as all three, like all seven of the young women, were accomplished tellers of stories with no fear whatever of Mrs. Grundy? And thus the "Decameron" of Giovanni Boccaccio came about.

S. Maria Novella also resembles S. Croce in its moving groups of sight-seers each in the hands of a guide. These one sees always and hears always: so much so that a reminder has been printed and set up here and there in this church, to the effect that it is primarily the house of God and for worshippers. But S. Maria Novella has not a tithe of S. Croce's treasures. Having almost no tombs of first importance, it has to rely upon its interior beauty and upon its frescoes, and its chief glory, whatever Mr. Ruskin, who hated them, might say, is, for most people, Ghirlandaio's series of scenes in the life of the Virgin and S. John the Baptist. These cover the walls of the choir and for more than four centuries have given delight to Florentines and foreigners. Such was the thoroughness of their painter in his colour mixing (in which the boy Michelangelo assisted him) that, although they have sadly dimmed and require the best morning light, they should endure for centuries longer, a reminder not only of the thoughtful sincere interesting art of Ghirlandaio and of the pious generosity of the Tornabuoni family, who gave them, but also of the costumes and carriage of the Florentine ladies at the end of the fifteenth century when Lorenzo the Magnificent was in his zenith. Domenico Ghirlandaio may not be quite of the highest rank among the makers of Florence; but he comes very near it, and indeed, by reason of being Michelangelo's first instructor, perhaps should stand amid them. But one thing is certain–that without him Florence would be the poorer by many beautiful works.

He was born in 1449, twenty-one years after the death of Masaccio and three before Leonardo, twenty-six before Michelangelo, and thirty-four before Raphael. His full name was Domenico or Tommaso di Currado di Doffo Bigordi, but his father Tommaso Bigordi, a goldsmith, having hit upon a peculiarly attractive way of making garlands for the hair, was known as Ghirlandaio, the garland maker; and time has effaced the Bigordi completely.

The portraits of both Tommaso and Domenico, side by side, occur in the fresco representing Joachim driven from the Temple: Domenico, who is to be seen second from the extreme right, a little resembles our Charles II. Like his father, and, as we have seen, like most of the artists of Florence, he too became a goldsmith, and his love of the jewels that goldsmiths made may be traced in his pictures; but at an early age he was sent to Alessio Baldovinetti to learn to be a painter. Alessio's work we find all over Florence: a Last Judgment in the Accademia, for example, but that is not a very pleasing thing; a Madonna Enthroned, in the Uffizi; the S. Miniato frescoes; the S. Trinità frescoes; and that extremely charming although faded work in the outer court of SS. Annunziata. For the most delightful picture from his hand, however, one has to go to the Louvre, where there is a Madonna and Child (1300 a), in the early Tuscan room, which has a charm not excelled by any such group that I know. The photographers still call it a Piero della Francesca, and the Louvre authorities omit to name it at all; but it is Alessio beyond question. Next it hangs the best Ghirlandaio that I know–the very beautiful Visitation, and, to add to the interest of this room to the returning Florentine wanderer, on the same wall are two far more attractive works by Bastiano Mainardi (Ghirlandaio's brother-in-law and assistant at S. Maria Novella) than any in Florence.

Alessio, who was born in 1427, was an open-handed ingenious man who could not only paint and do mosaic but once made a wonderful clock for Lorenzo. His experiments with colour were disastrous: hence most of his frescoes have perished; but possibly it was through Alessio's mistakes that Ghirlandaio acquired the use of such a lasting medium. Alessio was an independent man who painted from taste and not necessity.

Ghirlandaio's chief influences, however, were Masaccio, at the Carmine, Fra Lippo Lippi, and Verrocchio, who is thought also to have been Baldovinetti's pupil and whose Baptism of Christ, in the Accademia, painted when Ghirlandaio was seventeen, must have given Ghirlandaio the lines for his own treatment of the incident in this church. One has also only to compare Verrocchio's sculptured Madonnas in the Bargello with many of Ghirlandaio's to see the influence again; both were attracted by a similar type of sweet, easy-natured girl.

When he was twenty-six Ghirlandaio went to Rome to paint the Sixtine library, and then to San Gimignano, where he was assisted by Mainardi, who was to remain his most valuable ally in executing the large commissions which were to come to his workshop. His earliest Florentine frescoes are those which we shall see at Ognissanti; the Madonna della Misericordia and the Deposition painted for the Vespucci family and only recently discovered, together with the S. Jerome, in the church, and the Last Supper, in the refectory. By this time Ghirlandaio and Botticelli were in some sort of rivalry, although, so far as I know, friendly enough, and both went to Rome in 1481, together with Perugino, Piero di Cosimo, Cosimo Rosselli, Luca Signorelli and others, at the command of Pope Sixtus IV to decorate the Sixtine chapel, the excommunication of all Florentines which the Pope had decreed after the failure of the Pazzi Conspiracy to destroy the Medici (as we saw in chapter II) having been removed in order to get these excellent workmen to the Holy City. Painting very rapidly the little band had finished their work in six months, and Ghirlandaio was at home again with such an ambition and industry in him that he once expressed the wish that every inch of the walls of Florence might be covered by his brush–and in those days Florence had walls all round it, with twenty-odd towers in addition to the gates. His next great frescoes were those in the Palazzo Vecchio and S. Trinita. It was in 1485 that he painted his delightful Adoration, at the Accademia, and in 1486 he began his great series at S. Maria Novella, finishing them in 1490, his assistants being his brother David, Benedetto Mainardi, who married Ghirlandaio's sister, and certain apprentices, among them the youthful Michelangelo, who came to the studio in 1488.

The story of the frescoes is this. Ghirlandaio when in Rome had met Giovanni Tornabuoni, a wealthy merchant whose wife had died in childbirth. Her death we have already seen treated in relief by Verrocchio in the Bargello. Ghirlandaio was first asked to beautify in her honour the Minerva at Rome, where she was buried, and this he did. Later when Giovanni Tornabuoni wished to present S. Maria Novella with a handsome benefaction, he induced the Ricci family, who owned this chapel, to allow him to re-decorate it, and engaged Ghirlandaio for the task. This meant first covering the fast fading frescoes by Orcagna, which were already there, and then painting over them. What the Orcagnas were like we cannot know; but the substitute, although probably it had less of curious genius in it was undoubtedly more attractive to the ordinary observer.

The right wall, as one faces the window (whose richness of coloured glass, although so fine in the church as a whole, is here such a privation), is occupied by scenes in the story of the Baptist; the left by the life of the Virgin. The left of the lowest pair on the right wall represents S. Mary and S. Elizabeth, and in it a party of Ghirlandaio's stately Florentine ladies watch the greeting of the two saints outside Florence itself, symbolized rather than portrayed, very near the church in which we stand. The girl in yellow, on the right of the picture, with her handkerchief in her hand and wearing a rich dress, is Giovanna degli Albizzi, who married Lorenzo Tornabuoni at the Villa Lemmi near Florence, that villa from which Botticelli's exquisite fresco, now in the Louvre at the top of the main staircase, in which she again is to be seen, was taken. Her life was a sad one, for her husband was one of those who conspired with Piero di Lorenzo de' Medici for his return some ten years later, and was beheaded. S. Elizabeth is of course the older woman. The companion to this picture represents the angel appearing to S. Zacharias, and here again Ghirlandaio gives us contemporary Florentines, portraits of distinguished Tornabuoni men and certain friends of eminence among them. In the little group low down on the left, for example, are Poliziano and Marsilio Ficino, the Platonist. Above–but seeing is beginning to be difficult–the pair of frescoes represent, on the right, the birth of the Baptist, and on the left, his naming. The birth scene has much beauty, and is as well composed as any, and there is a girl in it of superb grace and nobility; but the birth scene of the Virgin, on the opposite wall, is perhaps the finer and certainly more easily seen. In the naming of the child we find Medici portraits once more, that family being related to the Tornabuoni; and Mr. Davies, in his book on Ghirlandaio, offers the interesting suggestion, which he supports very reasonably, that the painter has made the incident refer to the naming of Lorenzo de' Medici's third son, Giovanni (or John), who afterwards became Pope Leo X. In that case the man on the left, in green, with his hand on his hip, would be Lorenzo himself, whom he certainly resembles. Who the sponsor is is not known. The landscape and architecture are alike charming.

Above these we faintly see that strange Baptism of Christ, so curiously like the Verrocchio in the Accademia, and the Baptist preaching.

The left wall is perhaps the favourite. We begin with Joachim being driven from the Temple, one of the lowest pair; and this has a peculiar interest in giving us a portrait of the painter and his associates–the figure on the extreme right being Benedetto Mainardi; then Domenico Ghirlandaio; then his father; and lastly his brother David. On the opposite side of the picture is the fated Lorenzo Tornabuoni, of whom I have spoken above, the figure farthest from the edge, with his hand on his hip. The companion picture is the most popular of all–the Birth of the Virgin–certainly one of the most charming interiors in Florence. Here again we have portraits–no doubt Tornabuoni ladies–and much pleasant fancy on the part of the painter, who made everything as beautiful as he could, totally unmindful of the probabilities. Ruskin is angry with him for neglecting to show the splashing of the water in the vessel, but it would be quite possible for no splashing to be visible, especially if the pouring had only just begun; but for Ruskin's strictures you must go to "Mornings in Florence," where poor Ghirlandaio gets a lash for every virtue of Giotto. Next–above, on the left–we have the Presentation of the Virgin and on the right her Marriage. The Presentation is considered by Mr. Davies to be almost wholly the work of Ghirlandaio's assistants, while the youthful Michelangelo himself has been credited with the half-naked figure on the steps, although Mr. Davies gives it to Mainardi. Mainardi again is probably the author of the companion scene. The remaining frescoes are of less interest and much damaged; but in the window wall one should notice the portraits of Giovanni Tornabuoni and Francesca di Luca Pitti, his wife, kneeling, because this Giovanni was the donor of the frescoes, and his sister Lucrezia was the wife of Piero de' Medici and therefore the mother of Lorenzo the Magnificent, while Francesca Tornabuoni, the poor lady who died in childbirth, was the daughter of that proud Florentine who began the Pitti palace but ended his life in disgrace.

And so we leave this beautiful recess, where pure religious feeling may perhaps be wanting but where the best spirit of the Renaissance is to be found: everything making for harmony and pleasure; and on returning to London the visitor should make a point of seeing the Florentine girl by the same hand in our National Gallery, No. 1230, for she is very typical of his genius.

On the entrance wall of the church is what must once have been a fine Masaccio–"The Trinity"–but it is in very bad condition; while in the Cappella Rucellai in the right transept is what purports to be a Cimabue, very like the one in the Accademia, but with a rather more matured Child in it. Vasari tells us that on its completion this picture was carried in stately procession from the painter's studio to the church, in great rejoicing and blowing of trumpets, the populace being moved not only by religious ecstasy but by pride in an artist who could make such a beautiful and spacious painting, the largest then known. Vasari adds that when Cimabue was at work upon it, Charles of Anjou, visiting Florence, was taken to his studio, to see the wonderful painter, and a number of Florentines entering too, they broke out into such rejoicings that the locality was known ever after as Borgo Allegro, or Joyful Quarter. This would be about 1290. There was a certain fitness in Cimabue painting this Madonna, for it is said that he had his education in the convent which stood here before the present church was begun. But I should add that of Cimabue we know practically nothing, and that most of Vasari's statements have been confuted, while the painter of the S. Maria Novella Madonna is held by some authorities to be Duccio of Siena. So where are we?

The little chapel next the choir on the right is that of Filippo Strozzi the elder who was one of the witnesses of the Pazzi outrage in the Duomo in 1478. This was the Filippo Strozzi who began the Strozzi palace in 1489, father of the Filippo Strozzi who married Lorenzo de' Medici's noble granddaughter Clarice and came to a tragic end under Cosimo I. Old Filippo's tomb here was designed by Benedetto da Maiano, who made the famous Franciscan pulpit in S. Croce, and was Ghirlandaio's friend and the Strozzi palace's first architect. The beautiful circular relief of the Virgin and Child, with a border of roses and flying worshipping angels all about it, behind the altar, is Benedetto's too, and very lovely and human are both Mother and Child.

The frescoes in this chapel, by Filippino Lippi, are interesting, particularly that one on the left, depicting the Resuscitation of Drusiana by S. John the Evangelist, at Rome, in which the group of women and children on the right, with the little dog, is full of life and most naturally done. Above (but almost impossible to see) is S. John in his cauldron of boiling oil between Roman soldiers and the denouncing Emperor, under the banner S.P.Q.R.– a work in which Roman local colour completely excludes religious feeling. Opposite, below, we see S. Philip exorcising a dragon, a very florid scene, and, above, a painfully spirited and realistic representation of the Crucifixion. The sweetness of the figures of Charity and Faith in monochrome and gold helps, with Benedetto's tondo, to engentle the air.

We then come again to the Choir, with Ghirlandaio's urbane Florentine pageant in the guise of sacred history, and pass on to the next chapel, the Cappella Gondi, where that crucifix in wood is to be seen which Brunelleschi carved as a lesson to Donatello, who received it like the gentleman he was. I have told the story in Chapter XV.

The left transept ends in the chapel of the Strozzi family, of which Filippo was the head in his day, and here we find Andrea Orcagna and his brother's fresco of Heaven, the Last Judgment and Hell. It was the two Orcagnas who, according to Vasari, had covered the Choir with those scenes in the life of the Virgin which Ghirlandaio was allowed to paint over, and Vasari adds that the later artist availed himself of many of the ideas of his predecessors. This, however, is not very likely, I think, except perhaps in choice of subject. Orcagna, like Giotto, and later, Michelangelo, was a student of Dante, and the Strozzi chapel frescoes follow the poet's descriptions. In the Last Judgment, Dante himself is to be seen, among the elect, in the attitude of prayer. Petrarch is with him.

The sacristy is by Talenti (of the Campanile) and was added in 1350. Among its treasures once were the three reliquaries painted by Fra Angelico, but they are now at S. Marco. It has still rich vestments, fine woodwork, and a gay and elaborate lavabo by one of the della Robbias, with its wealth of ornament and colour and its charming Madonna and Child with angels.

A little doorway close by used to lead to the cloisters, and a mercenary sacristan was never far distant, only too ready to unlock for a fee what should never have been locked, and black with fury if he got nothing. But all this has now been done away with, and the entrance to the cloisters is from the Piazza, just to the left of the church, and there is a turnstile and a fee of fifty centimes. At S. Lorenzo the cloisters are free. At the Carmine and the Annunziata the cloisters are free. At S. Croce the charge is a lira and at S. Maria Novella half a lira. To make a charge for the cloisters alone seems to me utterly wicked. Let the Pazzi Chapel at S. Croce and the Spanish Chapel here have fees, if you like; but the cloisters should be open to all. Children should be encouraged to play there.

Since, however, S. Maria Novella imposes a fee we must pay it, and the new arrangement at any rate carries this advantage with it, that one knows what one is expected to pay and can count on entrance.

The cloisters are everywhere interesting to loiter in, but their chief fame is derived from the Spanish Chapel, which gained that name when in 1566 it was put at the disposal of Eleanor of Toledo's suite on the occasion of her marriage to Cosimo I. Nothing Spanish about it otherwise. Both structure and frescoes belong to the fourteenth century. Of these frescoes, which are of historical and human interest rather than artistically beautiful, that one on the right wall as we enter is the most famous. It is a pictorial glorification of the Dominican order triumphant; with a vivid reminder of the origin of the word Dominican in the episode of the wolves (or heretics) being attacked by black and white dogs, the Canes Domini, or hounds of the Lord. The "Mornings in Florence" should here be consulted again, for Ruskin made a very thorough and characteristically decisive analysis of these paintings, which, whether one agrees with it or not, is profoundly interesting. Poor old Vasari, who so patiently described them too and named a number of the originals of the portraits, is now shelved, and from both his artists, Simone Martini and Taddeo Gaddi, has the authorship been taken by modern experts. Some one, however, must have done the work. The Duomo as represented here is not the Duomo of fact, which had not then its dome, but of anticipation.

Opposite, we see a representation of the triumph of the greatest of the Dominicans, after its founder, S. Thomas Aquinas, the author of the "Summa Theologiae," who died in 1274. The painter shows the Angelic Doctor enthroned amid saints and patriarchs and heavenly attendants, while three powerful heretics grovel at his feet, and beneath are the Sciences and Moral Qualities and certain distinguished men who served them conspicuously, such as Aristotle, the logician, whom S. Thomas Aquinas edited, and Cicero, the rhetorician. In real life Aquinas was so modest and retiring that he would accept no exalted post from the Church, but remained closeted with his books and scholars; and we can conceive what his horror would be could he view this apotheosis. On the ceiling is a quaint rendering of the walking on the water, S. Peter's failure being watched from the ship with the utmost closeness by the other disciples, but attracting no notice whatever from an angler, close by, on the shore. The chapel is desolate and unkempt, and those of us who are not Dominicans are not sorry to leave it and look for the simple sweetness of the Giottos.

These are to be found, with some difficulty, on the walls of the niche where the tomb of the Marchese Ridolfo stands. They are certainly very simple and telling, and I advise every one to open the "Mornings in Florence" and learn how the wilful magical pen deals with them; but it would be a pity to give up Ghirlandaio because Giotto was so different, as Ruskin wished. Room for both. One scene represents the meeting of S. Joachim and S. Anna outside a mediaeval city's walls, and it has some pretty Giottesque touches, such as the man carrying doves to the Temple and the angel uniting the two saints in friendliness; and the other is the Birth of the Virgin, which Ruskin was so pleased to pit against Ghirlandaio's treatment of the same incident. Well, it is given to some of us to see only what we want to see and be blind to the rest; and Ruskin was of these the very king. I agree with him that Ghirlandaio in both his Nativity frescoes thought little of the exhaustion of the mothers; but it is arguable that two such accouchements might with propriety be treated as abnormal–as indeed every painter has treated the birth of Christ, where the Virgin, fully dressed, is receiving the Magi a few moments after. Ruskin, after making his deadly comparisons, concludes thus genially of the Giotto version–"If you can be pleased with this, you can see Florence. But if not, by all means amuse yourself there, if you can find it amusing, as long as you like; you can never see it."

The S. Maria Novella habit is one to be quickly contracted by the visitor to Florence: nearly as important as the S. Croce habit. Both churches are hospitable and, apart from the cloisters, free and eminently suited for dallying in; thus differing from the Duomo, which is dark, and S. Lorenzo, where there are payments to be made and attendants to discourage.

An effort should be made at S. Maria Novella to get into the old cloisters, which are very large and indicate what a vast convent it once was. But there is no certainty. The way is to go through to the Palaestra and hope for the best. Here, as I have said in the second chapter, were lodged Pope Eugenius and his suite, when they came to the Council of Florence in 1439. These large and beautiful green cloisters are now deserted. Through certain windows on the left one may see chemists at work compounding drugs and perfumes after old Dominican recipes, to be sold at the Farmacia in the Via della Scala close by. The great refectory has been turned into a gymnasium.

The two obelisks, supported by tortoises and surmounted by beautiful lilies, in the Piazza of S. Maria Novella were used as boundaries in the chariot races held here under Cosimo I, and in the collection of old Florentine prints on the top floor of Michelangelo's house you may see representations of these races. The charming loggia opposite S. Maria Novella, with della Robbia decorations, is the Loggia di S. Paolo, a school designed, it is thought, by Brunelleschi, and here, at the right hand end, we see S. Dominic himself in a friendly embrace with S. Francis, a very beautiful group by either Luca or Andrea della Robbia.

In the loggia cabmen now wrangle all day and all night. From it S. Maria Novella is seen under the best conditions, always cheerful and serene; while far behind the church is the huge Apennine where most of the weather of Florence seems to be manufactured. In mid April this year (1912) it still had its cap of snow.

CHAPTER XXII

THE Piazza Vittorio Emmanuele to S. Trinità

A city of trams–The old market–Donatello's figure of Abundance–An evening resort–A hall of variety–Florentines of to-day–The war with Turkey–Homecoming heroes–Restaurants–The new market–The bronze boar–A fifteenth century palace–Old Florentine life reconstructed–Where changes are few–S. Trinità–Ghirlandaio again–S. Francis–The Strozzi palace–Clarice de' Medici.

Florence is not simple to the stranger. Like all very old cities built fortuitously it is difficult to learn: the points of the compass are elusive; the streets are so narrow that the sky is no constant guide; the names of the streets are often not there; the policemen have no high standard of helpfulness. There are trams, it is true–too many and too noisy, and too near the pavement–but the names of their outward destinations, from the centre, too rarely correspond to any point of interest that one is desiring. Hence one has many embarrassments and even annoyances. Yet I daresay this is best: an orderly Florence is unthinkable. Since, however, the trams that are returning to the centre nearly all go to the Duomo, either passing it or stopping there, the tram becomes one's best friend and the Duomo one's starting point for most excursions.

Supposing ourselves to be there once more, let us quickly get through the horrid necessity, which confronts one in all ancient Italian cities, of seeing the Piazza Vittorio Emmanuele. In an earlier chapter we left the Baptistery and walked along the Via Calzaioli. Again starting from the Baptistery let us take the Via dell' Arcivescovado, which is parallel with the Via Calzaioli, on the right of it, and again walk straight forward. We shall come almost at once to the great modern square.

No Italian city or town is complete without a Piazza Vittorio Emmanuele and a statue of that monarch. In Florence the sturdy king bestrides his horse here. Italy being so old and Vittorio Emmanuele so new, it follows in most cases that the square or street named after him supplants an older one, and if the Italians had any memory or imaginative interest in history they would see to it that the old name was not wholly obliterated. In Florence, in order to honour the first king of United Italy, much grave violence was done to antiquity, for a very picturesque quarter had to be cleared away for the huge brasseries, stores and hotels which make up the west side; which in their turn marked the site of the old market where Donatello and Brunelleschi and all the later artists of the great days did their shopping and met to exchange ideals and banter; and that market in its turn marked the site of the Roman forum.

One of the features of the old market was the charming Loggia di Pesce; another, Donatello's figure of Abundance, surmounting a column. This figure is now in the museum of ancient city relics in the monastery of S. Marco, where one confronts her on a level instead of looking up at her in mid sky. But she is very good, none the less.

In talking to elderly persons who can remember Florence forty and fifty years ago I find that nothing so distresses them as the loss of the old quarter for the making of this new spacious piazza; and probably nothing can so delight the younger Florentines as its possession, for, having nothing to do in the evenings, they do it chiefly in the Piazza Vittorio Emmanuele. Chairs and tables spring up like mushrooms in the roadway, among which too few waiters distribute those very inexpensive refreshments which seem to be purchased rather for the right to the seat that they confer than for any stimulation. It is extraordinary to the eyes of the thriftless English, who are never so happy as when they are overpaying Italian and other caterers in their own country, to notice how long these wiser folk will occupy a table on an expenditure of fourpence.

I do not mean that there are no theatres in Florence. There are many, but they are not very good; and the young men can do without them. Curious old theatres, faded and artificial, all apparently built for the comedies of Goldoni. There are cinema theatres too, at prices which would delight the English public addicted to those insidious entertainments, but horrify English managers; and the Teatro Salvini at the back of the Palazzo Vecchio is occasionally transformed into a Folies Bergères (as it is called) where one after another comediennes sing each two or three songs rapidly to an audience who regard them with apathy and converse without ceasing. The only sign of interest which one observes is the murmur which follows anything a little off the beaten track–a sound that might equally be encouragement or disapproval. But a really pretty woman entering a box moves them. Then they employ every note in the gamut; and curiously enough the pretty woman in the box is usually as cool under the fusillade as a professional and hardened sister would be. A strange music hall this to the English eye, where the orchestra smokes, and no numbers are put up, and every one talks, and the intervals seem to be hours long. But the Florentines do not mind, for they have not the English thirst for entertainment and escape; they carry their entertainment with them and do not wish to escape–going to such places only because they are warmer than out of doors.

Sitting here and watching their ironical negligence of the stage and their interest in each other's company; their animated talk and rapid decisions as to the merits and charms of a performer; the comfort of their attitudes and carelessness (although never quite slovenliness) in dress; one seems to realize the nation better than anywhere. The old fighting passion may have gone;

but much of the quickness, the shrewdness and the humour remains, together with the determination of each man to have if possible his own way and, whether possible or not, his own say.

Seeing them in great numbers one quickly learns and steadily corroborates the fact that the Florentines are not beautiful. A pretty woman or a handsome man is a rarity; but a dull-looking man or woman is equally rare. They are shrewd, philosophic, cynical, and very ready for laughter. They look contented also: Florence clearly is the best place to be born in, to live in, and to die in. Let all the world come to Florence, by all means, and spend its money there; but don't ask Florence to go to the world. Don't in fact ask Florence to do anything very much.

Civilization and modern conditions have done the Florentines no good. Their destiny was to live in a walled city in turbulent days, when the foe came against it, or tyranny threatened from within and had to be resisted. They were then Florentines and everything mattered. To-day they are Italians and nothing matters very much. Moreover, it must be galling to have somewhere in the recesses of their consciousness the knowledge that their famous city, built and cemented with their ancestors' blood, is now only a museum.

When it is fine and warm the music hall does not exist, and it is in the Piazza Vittorio Emmanuele that the Florentines sit and talk, or walk and talk, or listen to the band which periodically inhabits a stand near the centre; and it was here that I watched the reception of the news that Italy had declared war on Turkey, a decision which while it rejoiced the national warlike spirit of the populace could not but carry with it a reminder that wars have to be paid for. Six or seven months later I saw the return to Florence of the first troops from the war, and their reception was terrific. In the mass they were welcome enough; but as soon as units could be separated from the mass the fun began, for they were carried shoulder high to whatever destination they wanted, their knapsacks and rifles falling to proud bearers too; while the women clapped from the upper windows, the shrewd shopkeepers cheered from their doorways, and the crowd which followed and surrounded the hero every moment increased. As for the heroes, they looked for the most part a good deal less foolish than Englishmen would have done; but here and there was one whose expression suggested that the Turks were nothing to this. One poor fellow had his coat dragged from his back and torn into a thousand souvenirs.

The restaurants of Florence are those of a city where the natives are thrifty and the visitors dine in hotels. There is one expensive high-class house, in the Via Tornabuoni–Doney e Nipoti or Doney et Neveux–where the cooking is Franco-Italian, and the Chianti and wines are dear beyond belief, and the venerable waiters move with a deliberation which can drive a hungry man–and one is always hungry in this fine Tuscan air–to despair. I like better the excellent old-fashioned purely Italian food and Chianti and speed at Bonciani's in the Via de Panzani, close to the station. These twain are the best. But it is more interesting to go to the huge Gambrinus in the Piazza Vittorio Emmanuele, because so much is going on all the time. One curious Florentine habit is quickly discovered and resented by the stranger who frequents a restaurant, and that is the system of changing waiters from one set of tables to another; so that whereas in London and Paris the wise diner is true to a corner because it carries the same service with it, in Florence he must follow the service. But if the restaurants have odd ways, and a limited range of dishes and those not very interesting, they make up for it by being astonishingly quick. Things are cooked almost miraculously.

The Florentines eat little. But greediness is not an Italian fault. No greedy people would have a five-syllabled word for waiter.

Continuing along the Via dell' Arcivescovado, which after the Piazza becomes the Via Celimana, we come to that very beautiful structure the Mercato Nuovo, which, however, is not so wonderfully new, having been built as long ago as 1547-1551. Its columns and arched roof are exquisitely proportioned. As a market it seems to be a poor affair, the chief commodity being straw hats. For the principal food market one has to go to the Via d'Ariento, near S. Lorenzo, and this is, I think, well worth doing early in the morning. Lovers of Hans Andersen go to the Mercato Nuovo to see the famous bronze boar (or "metal pig," as it was called in the translation on which I was brought up) that stands here, on whose back the little street boy had such adventures. The boar himself was the work of Pietro Tacca (1586-1650), a copy from an ancient marble original, now in the Uffizi, at the top of the entrance stairs; but the pedestal with its collection of creeping things is modern. The Florentines who stand in the market niches are Bernardo Cennini, a goldsmith and one of Ghiberti's assistants, who introduced printing into Florence in 1471 and began with an edition of Virgil; Giovanni Villani, who was the city's first serious historian, beginning in 1300 and continuing till his death in 1348; and Michele Lando, the wool-carder, who on July 22nd, 1378, at the head of a mob, overturned the power of the Signory.

By continuing straight on we should come to that crowded and fussy little street which crosses the river by the Ponte Vecchio and eventually becomes the Roman way; but let us instead turn to the right this side of the market, down the Via Porta Rossa, because here is the Palazzo Davanzati, which has a profound interest to lovers of the Florentine past in that it has been restored exactly to its ancient state when Pope Eugenius IV lodged here, and has been filled with fourteenth and fifteenth century furniture. In those days it was the home of the Davizza family. The Davanzati bought it late in the sixteenth century and retained it until 1838. In 1904 it was bought by Professor Elia Volpi, who restored its ancient conditions and presented it to the city as a permanent monument of the past.

Here we see a mediaeval Florentine palace precisely as it was when its Florentine owner lived his uncomfortable life there. For say what one may, there is no question that life must have been uncomfortable. In early and late summer, when the weather was fine and warm, these stone floors and continuous draughts may have been solacing; but in winter and early spring, when Florentine weather can be so bitterly hostile, what then? That there was a big fire we know by the smoky condition of Michelozzo's charming frieze on the chimney piece; but the room–I refer to that on the first floor–is so vast that this fire can have done little for any one but an immediate vis-à-vis; and the room, moreover, was between the open world on the one side, and the open court (now roofed in with glass) on the other, with such additional opportunities for draughts as the four trap-doors in the floor offered. It was through these traps that the stone cannon-balls still stacked in the window seats were dropped, or a few gallons of boiling oil poured, whenever the city or a faction of it turned against the householder. Not comfortable, you see, at least not in our northern sense of the word, although to the hardy frugal Florentine it may have seemed a haven of luxury.

The furniture of the salon is simple and sparse and very hard. A bust here, a picture there, a coloured plate, a crucifix, and a Madonna and Child in a niche: that was all the decoration save tapestry. An hour glass, a pepper mill, a compass, an inkstand, stand for utility, and quaint and twisted musical instruments and a backgammon board for beguilement.

In the salle-à-manger adjoining is less light, and here also is a symbol of Florentine unrest in the shape of a hole in the wall (beneath the niche which holds the Madonna and Child) through which the advancing foe, who had successfully avoided the cannon balls and the oil, might be prodded with lances, or even fired at. The next room is the kitchen, curiously far from the well, the opening to which is in the salon, and then a bedroom (with some guns in it) and smaller rooms gained from the central court.

The rest of the building is the same–a series of self-contained flats, but all dipping for water from the same shaft and all depending anxiously upon the success of the first floor with invaders. At the top is a beautiful loggia with Florence beneath it.

The odd thing to remember is that for the poor of Florence, who now inhabit houses of the same age as the Davanzati palace, the conditions are almost as they were in the fifteenth century. A few changes have come in, but hardly any. Myriads of the tenements have no water laid on: it must still be pulled up in buckets exactly as here. Indeed you may often see the top floor at work in this way; and there is a row of houses on the left of the road to the Certosa, a little way out of Florence, with a most elaborate network of bucket ropes over many gardens to one well. Similarly one sees the occupants of the higher floors drawing vegetables and bread in baskets from the street and lowering the money for them. The postman delivers letters in this way, too. Again, one of the survivals of the Davanzati to which the custodian draws attention is the rain-water pipe, like a long bamboo, down the wall of the court; but one has but to walk along the Via Lambertesca, between the Uffizi and the Via Por S. Maria, and peer into the alleys, to see that these pipes are common enough yet.

In fact, directly one leaves the big streets Florence is still fifteenth century. Less colour in the costumes, and a few anachronisms, such as gas or electric light, posters, newspapers, cigarettes, and bicycles, which dart like dragon flies (every Florentine cyclist being a trick cyclist); but for the rest there is no change. The business of life has not altered; the same food is eaten, the same vessels contain it, the same fire cooks it, the same red wine is made from the same grapes in the same vineyards, the same language (almost) is spoken. The babies are christened at the same font, the parents visit the same churches. Similarly the handicrafts can have altered little. The coppersmith, the blacksmith, the cobbler, the woodcarver, the goldsmiths in their yellow smocks, must be just as they were, and certainly the cellars and caverns under the big houses in which they work have not changed. Where the change is, is among the better-to-do, the rich, and in the government. For no longer is a man afraid to talk freely of politics; no longer does he shudder as he passes the Bargello; no longer is the name of Medici on his lips. Everything else is practically as it was.

The Via Porta Rossa runs to the Piazza S. Trinità, the church of S. Trinità being our destination. For here are some interesting frescoes. First, however, let us look at the sculpture: a very beautiful altar by Benedetto da Rovezzano in the fifth chapel of the right aisle; a monument by Luca della Robbia to one of the archbishops of Fiesole, once in S. Pancrazio (which is now a tobacco factory) in the Via della Spada and brought here for safe keeping–a beautiful example of Luca's genius, not only as a modeller but also as a very treasury of pretty thoughts, for the border of flowers and leaves is beyond praise delightful. The best green in Florence (after Nature's, which is seen through so many doorways and which splashes over so many white walls and mingles with gay fruits in so many shops) is here.

In the fifth chapel of the left aisle is a Magdalen carved in wood by Desiderio da Settignano and finished by Benedetto da Maiano; while S. Trinità now possesses, but shows only on Good Friday, the very crucifix from S. Miniato which bowed down and blessed S. Gualberto. The porphyry tombs of the Sassetti, in the chapel of that family, by Giuliano di Sangallo, are magnificent.

It is in the Sassetti chapel that we find the Ghirlandaio frescoes of scenes in the life of S. Francis which bring so many strangers to this church. The painting which depicts S. Francis receiving the charter from the Emperor Honorius is interesting both for its history and its painting; for it contains a valuable record of what the Palazzo Vecchio and Loggia de' Lanzi were like in 1485, and also many portraits: among them Lorenzo the Magnificent, on the extreme right holding out his hand: Poliziano, tutor of the Medici boys, coming first up the stairs; and on the extreme left very probably Verrocchio, one of Ghirlandaio's favourite painters. We find old Florence again in the very attractive picture of the resuscitation of the nice little girl in violet, a daughter of the Spini family, who fell from a window of the Spini palace (as we see in the distance on the left, this being one of the old synchronized scenes) and was brought to life by S. Francis, who chanced to be flying by. The scene is intensely local: just outside the church, looking along what is now the Piazza S. Trinità and the old Trinità bridge. The Spini palace is still there, but is now called the Ferroni, and it accommodates no longer Florentine aristocrats but consuls and bank clerks. Among the portraits in the fresco are noble friends of the Spini family–Albrizzi, Acciaioli, Strozzi and so forth. The little girl is very quaint and perfectly ready to take up once more the threads of her life. How long she lived this second time and what became of her I have not been able to discover. Her tiny sister, behind the bier, is even quainter. On the left is a little group of the comely Florentine ladies in whom Ghirlandaio so delighted, tall and serene, with a few youths among them.

It is interesting to note that Ghirlandaio in his S. Trinità frescoes and Benedetto da Maiano in his S. Croce pulpit reliefs chose exactly the same scenes in the life of S. Francis: interesting because when Ghirlandaio was painting frescoes at San Gimignano in 1475, Benedetto was at work on the altar for the same church of S. Fina, and they were friends. Where Ghirlandaio and Giotto, also in S. Croce, also coincide in choice of subject some interesting comparisons may be made, all to the advantage of Giotto in spiritual feeling and unsophisticated charm, but by no means to Ghirlandaio's detriment as a fascinating historian in colour. In the scene of the death of S. Francis we find Ghirlandaio and Giotto again on the same ground, and here it is probable that the later painter went to the earlier for inspiration; for he has followed Giotto in the fine thought that makes one of the attendant brothers glance up as though at the saint's ascending spirit. It is remarkable how, with every picture that one sees, Giotto's completeness of equipment as a religious painter becomes more marked. His hand may have been ignorant of many masterly devices for which the time was not ripe; but his head and heart knew all.

The patriarchs in the spandrels of the choir are by Ghirlandaio's master, Alessio Baldovinetti, of whom I said something in the chapter on S. Maria Novella. They once more testify to this painter's charm and brilliance. Almost more than that of any other does one regret the scarcity of his work. It was fitting that he should have painted the choir, for his name-saint, S. Alessio, guards the façade of the church.

The column opposite the church came from the baths of Caracalla and was set up by Cosimo I, upon the attainment of his life-long ambition of a grand-dukeship and a crown. The figure at the top is Justice.

S. Trinità is a good starting-point for the leisurely examination of the older and narrower streets, an occupation which so many visitors to Florence prefer to the study of picture galleries and churches. And perhaps rightly. In no city can they carry on their researches with such ease, for Florence is incurious about them. Either the Florentines are too much engrossed in their own affairs or the peering foreigner has become too familiar an object to merit notice, but one may drift about even in the narrowest alleys beside the Arno, east and west, and attract few eyes. And the city here is at its most romantic: between the Piazza S. Trinità and the Via Por S. Maria, all about the Borgo SS. Apostoli.

We have just been discussing Benedetto da Maiano the sculptor. If we turn to the left on leaving S. Trinità, instead of losing ourselves in the little streets, we are in the Via Tornabuoni, where the best shops are and American is the prevailing language. We shall soon come, on the right, to an example of Benedetto's work as an architect, for the first draft of the famous Palazzo Strozzi, the four-square fortress-home which Filippo Strozzi began for himself in 1489, was his. Benedetto continued the work until his death in 1507, when Cronaca, who built the great hall in the Palazzo Vecchio, took it over and added the famous cornice. The iron lantern and other smithwork were by Lorenzo the Magnificent's sardonic friend, "Il Caparro," of the Sign of the Burning Books, of whom I wrote in the chapter on the Medici palace.

The first mistress of the Strozzi palace was Clarice Strozzi, née Clarice de' Medici, the daughter of Piero, son of Lorenzo the Magnificent. She was born in 1493 and married Filippo Strozzi the younger in 1508, during the family's second period of exile. They then lived at Rome, but were allowed to return to Florence in 1510. Clarice's chief title to fame is her proud outburst when she turned Ippolito and Alessandro out of the Medici palace. She died in 1528 and was buried in S. Maria Novella. The unfortunate Filippo met his end nine years later in the Boboli fortezza, which his money had helped to build and in which he was imprisoned for his share in a conspiracy against Cosimo I. Cosimo confiscated the palace and all Strozzi's other possessions, but later made some restitution. To-day the family occupy the upper part of their famous imperishable home, and beneath there is an exhibition of pictures and antiquities for sale. No private individual, whatever his wealth or ambition, will probably ever again succeed in building a house half so strong or noble as this.

CHAPTER XXIII

THE Pitti

Luca Pitti's pride–Preliminary caution–A terrace view–A collection but not a gallery–The personally-conducted–Giorgione the superb–Sustermans–The "Madonna del Granduca"–The "Madonna della Sedia"–From Cimabue to Raphael–Andrea del Sarto–Two Popes and a bastard–The ill-fated Ippolito–The National Gallery–Royal apartments–"Pallas Subduing the Centaur"–The Boboli Gardens.

The Pitti approached from the Via Guicciardini is far liker a prison than a palace. It was commissioned by Luca Pitti, one of the proudest and richest of the rivals of the Medici, in 1441. Cosimo de' Medici, as we have seen, had rejected Brunelleschi's plans for a palazzo as being too pretentious and gone instead to his friend Michelozzo for something that externally at any rate was more modest; Pitti, whose one ambition was to exceed Cosimo in power, popularity, and visible wealth, deliberately chose Brunelleschi, and gave him carte blanche to make the most magnificent mansion possible. Pitti, however, plotting against Cosimo's son Piero, was frustrated and condemned to death; and although Piero obtained his pardon he lost all his friends and passed into utter disrespect in the city. Meanwhile his palace remained unfinished and neglected, and continued so for a century, when it was acquired by the Grand Duchess Eleanor of Toledo, the wife of Cosimo I, who though she saw only the beginnings of its splendours lived there awhile and there brought up her doomed brood. Eleanor's architect–or rather Cosimo's, for though the Grand Duchess paid, the Grand Duke controlled–was Ammanati, the designer of the Neptune fountain in the Piazza della Signoria. Other important additions were made later. The last Medicean Grand Duke to occupy the Pitti was Gian Gastone, a bizarre detrimental, whose head, in a monstrous wig, may be seen at the top of the stairs leading to the Uffizi gallery. He died in 1737.

As I have said in chapter VIII, it was by the will of Gian Gastone's sister, widow of the Elector Palatine, who died in 1743, that the Medicean collections became the property of the Florentines. This bequest did not, however, prevent the migration of many of the best pictures to Paris under Napoleon, but after Waterloo they came back. The Pitti continued to be the home of princes after Gian Gastone quitted a world which he found strange and made more so; but they were not of the Medici blood. It is now a residence of the royal family.

The first thing to do if by evil chance one enters the Pitti by the covered way from the Uffizi is, just before emerging into the palace, to avoid the room where copies of pictures are sold, for not only is it a very catacomb of headache, from the fresh paint, but the copies are in themselves horrible and lead to disquieting reflections on the subject of sweated labour. The next thing to do, on at last emerging, is to walk out on the roof from the little room at the top of the stairs, and get a supply of fresh air for the gallery, and see Florence, which is very beautiful from here. Looking over the city one notices that the tower of the Palazzo Vecchio is almost more dominating than the Duomo, the work of the same architect who began this palace. Between the two is Fiesole. The Signoria tower is, as I say, the highest. Then the Duomo. Then Giotto's Campanile. The Bargello is hidden, but the graceful Badia tower is seen; also the little white Baptistery roof with its lantern just showing. From the fortezza come the sounds of drums and bugles.

Returning from this terrace we skirt a vast porphyry basin and reach the top landing of the stairs (which was, I presume, once a loggia) where there is a very charming marble fountain; and from this we enter the first room of the gallery. The Pitti walls are so congested and so many of the pictures so difficult to see, that I propose to refer only to those which, after a series of visits, seem to me the absolute best. Let me hasten to say that to visit the Pitti gallery on any but a really bright day is folly. The great windows (which were to be larger than Cosimo de' Medici's doors) are excellent to look out of, but the rooms are so crowded with paintings on walls and ceilings, and the curtains are so absorbent of light, that unless there is sunshine one gropes in gloom. The only pictures in short that are properly visible are those on screens or hinges; and these are, fortunately almost without exception, the best. The Pitti rooms were never made for pictures at all, and it is really absurd that so many beautiful things should be massed here without reasonable lighting.

The Pitti also is always crowded. The Uffizi is never crowded; the Accademia is always comfortable; the Bargello is sparsely attended. But the Pitti is normally congested, not only by individuals but by flocks, whose guides, speaking broken English, and sometimes broken American, lead from room to room. I need hardly say that they form the tightest knots before the works of Raphael. All this is proper enough, of course, but it serves to render the Pitti a difficult gallery rightly to study pictures in.

In the first chapter on the Uffizi I have said how simple it is, in the Pitti, to name the best picture of all, and how difficult in most galleries. But the Pitti has one particular jewel which throws everything into the background: the work not of a Florentine but of a Venetian: "The Concert" of Giorgione, which stands on an easel in the Sala di Marte. [9] It is true that modern criticism has doubted the lightness of the ascription, and many critics, whose one idea seems to be to deprive Giorgione of any pictures at all, leaving him but a glorious name without anything to account for it, call it an early Titian;

but this need not trouble us. There the picture is, and never do I think to see anything more satisfying. Piece by piece, it is not more than fine rich painting, but as a whole it is impressive and mysterious and enchanting. Pater compares the effect of it to music; and he is right.

The Sala dell' Iliade (the name of each room refers always to the ceiling painting, which, however, one quite easily forgets to look at) is chiefly notable for the Raphael just inside the door: "La Donna Gravida," No. 229, one of his more realistic works, with bolder colour than usual and harder treatment; rather like the picture that has been made its pendant, No. 224, an "Incognita" by Ridolfo Ghirlandaio, very firmly painted, but harder still. Between them is the first of the many Pitti Andrea del Sartos: No. 225, an "Assumption of the Madonna," opposite a similar work from the same brush, neither containing quite the finest traits of this artist. But the youth with outstretched hand at the tomb is nobly done. No. 265, "Principe Mathias de' Medici," is a good bold Sustermans, but No. 190, on the opposite wall, is a far better–a most charming work representing the Crown Prince of Denmark, son of Frederick III. Justus Sustermans, who has so many portraits here and elsewhere in Florence, was a Belgian, born in 1597, who settled in Florence as a portrait painter to Cosimo III. Van Dyck greatly admired his work and painted him. He died at Florence in 1681.

No. 208, a "Virgin Enthroned," by Fra Bartolommeo, is from S. Marco, and it had better have been painted on the wall there, like the Fra Angelicos, and then the convent would have it still. The Child is very attractive, as almost always in this artist's work, but the picture as a whole has grown rather dingy. By the window is a Velasquez, the first we have seen in Florence, a little Philip IV on his prancing steed, rather too small for its subject, but very interesting here among the Italians.

In the next large room–the Sala di Saturno–we come again to Raphael, who is indeed the chief master of the Pitti, his exquisite "Madonna del Granduca" being just to the left of the door. Here we have the simplest colouring and perfect sweetness, and such serenity of mastery as must be the despair of the copyists, who, however, never cease attempting it. The only defect is a little clumsiness in the Madonna's hand. The picture was lost for two centuries and it then changed owners for twelve crowns, the seller being a poor woman and the buyer a bookseller. The bookseller found a ready purchaser in the director of the Grand Duke Ferdinand III's gallery, and the Grand Duke so esteemed it that he carried it with him on all his journeys, just as Sir George Beaumont, the English connoisseur, never travelled without a favourite Claude. Hence its name. Another Andrea del Sarto, the "Disputa sulla Trinita," No. 172, is close by, nobly drawn but again not of his absolute best, and then five more Raphaels or putative Raphaels–No. 171, Tommaso Inghirami; No. 61, Angelo Doni, the collector and the friend of artists, for whom Michelangelo painted his "Holy Family" in the Uffizi; No. 59, Maddalena Doni; and above all No. 174, "The Vision of Ezekiel," that little great picture, so strong and spirited, and–to coin a word–Sixtinish. All these, I may say, are questioned by experts; but some very fine hand is to be seen in them any way. Over the "Ezekiel" is still another, No. 165, the "Madonna detta del Baldacchino," which is so much better in the photographs. Next this group–No. 164–we find Raphael's friend Perugino with an Entombment, but it lacks his divine glow; and above it a soft and mellow and easy Andrea del Sarto, No. 163, which ought to be in a church rather than here. A better Perugino is No. 42, which has all his sweetness, but to call it the Magdalen is surely wrong; and close by it a rather formal Fra Bartolommeo, No. 159, "Gesu Resuscitato," from the church of SS. Annunziata, in which once again the babies who hold the circular landscape are the best part. After another doubtful Raphael–the sly Cardinal Divizio da Bibbiena, No. 158–let us look at an unquestioned one, No. 151, the most popular picture in Florence, if not the whole world, Raphael's "Madonna della Sedia," that beautiful rich scene of maternal tenderness and infantine peace. Personally I do not find myself often under Raphael's spell; but here he conquers. The Madonna again is without enough expression, but her arms are right, and the Child is right, and the colour is so rich, almost Venetian in that odd way in which Raphael now and then could suggest Venice.

It is interesting to compare Raphael's two famous Madonnas in this room: this one belonging to his Roman period and the other, opposite it, to Florence, with the differences so marked. For by the time he painted this he knew more of life and human affection. This picture, I suppose, might be called the consummation of Renaissance painting in fullest bloom: the latest triumph of that impulse. I do not say it is the best; but it may be called a crown on the whole movement both in subject and treatment. Think of the gulf between the Cimabue Madonna and the Giotto Madonna, side by side, which we saw in the Accademia, and this. With so many vivid sympathies Giotto must have wanted with all his soul to make the mother motherly and the child childlike; but the time was not yet; his hand was neither free nor fit. Between Giotto and Raphael had to come many things before such treatment as this was possible; most of all, I think, Luca della Robbia had to come between, for he was the most valuable reconciler of God and man of them all. He was the first to bring a tender humanity into the Church, the first to know that a mother's fingers, holding a baby, sink into its soft little body. Without Luca I doubt if the "Madonna della Sedia" could be the idyll of protective solicitude and loving pride that it is.

The Sala di Giove brings us to Venetian painting indeed, and glorious painting too, for next the door is Titian's "Bella," No. 18, the lady in the peacock-blue dress with purple sleeves, all richly embroidered in gold, whom to see once is to remember for ever. On the other side of the door is Andrea's brilliant "S. John the Baptist as a Boy," No. 272, and then the noblest Fra Bartolommeo here, a Deposition, No. 64, not good in colour, but superbly drawn and pitiful. In this room also is the monk's great spirited figure of S. Marco, for the convent of that name. Between them is a Tintoretto, No. 131, Vincenzo Zeino, one of his ruddy old men, with a glimpse of Venice, under an angry sky, through the window. Over the door, No. 124, is an Annunciation by Andrea, with a slight variation in it, for two angels accompany that one who brings the news, and the announcement is made from the right instead of the left, while the incident is being watched by some people on the terrace over a classical portico. A greater Andrea hangs next: No. 123, the Madonna in Glory, fine but rather formal, and, like all Andrea's work, hallmarked by its woman type. The other notable pictures are Raphael's Fornarina, No. 245, which is far more Venetian than the "Madonna della Sedia," and has been given to Sebastian del Piombo; and the Venetian group on the right of the door, which is not only interesting for its own charm but as being a foretaste of the superb and glorious Giorgione in the Sala di Marte, which we now enter.

Here we find a Rembrandt, No. 16, an old man: age and dignity emerging golden from the gloom; and as a pendant a portrait, with somewhat similar characteristics, but softer, by Tintoretto, No. 83. Between them is a prosperous, ruddy group of scholars by Rubens, who has placed a vase of tulips before the bust of Seneca. And we find Rubens again with a sprawling, brilliant feat entitled "The Consequences of War," but what those consequences are, beyond nakedness, one has difficulty in discerning. Raphael's Holy Family, No. 94 (also known as the "Madonna dell' Impannata"), next it might be called the perfection of drawing without feeling. The authorities consider it a school piece: that is to say, chiefly the work of his imitators. The vivacity of the Child's face is very remarkable. The best Andrea is in this room–a Holy Family, No. 81, which gets sweeter and simpler and richer with every glance. Other Andreas are here too, notably on the right of the further door a sweet mother and sprawling, vigorous Child. But every Andrea that I see makes me think more highly of the "Madonna della Sacco," in the cloisters of SS. Annunziata. Van Dyck, who painted much in Italy before settling down at the English court, we find in this room with a masterly full-length seated portrait of an astute cardinal. But the room's greatest glory, as I have said, is the Giorgione on the easel.

In the Sala di Apollo, at the right of the door as we enter, is Andrea's portrait of himself, a serious and mysterious face shining out of darkness, and below it is Titian's golden Magdalen, No. 67, the same ripe creature that we saw at the Uffizi posing as Flora, again diffusing Venetian light. On the other side of the door we find, for the first time in Florence, Murillo, who has two groups of the Madonna and Child on this wall, the better being No. 63, which is both sweet and masterly. In No. 56 the Child becomes a pretty Spanish boy playing with a rosary, and in both He has a faint nimbus instead of the halo to which we are accustomed. On the same wall is another fine Andrea, who is most lavishly represented in this gallery, No. 58, a Deposition, all gentle melancholy rather than grief. The kneeling girl is very beautiful.

Finally there are Van Dyck's very charming portrait of Charles I of England and Henrietta, a most deft and distinguished work, and Raphael's famous portrait of Leo X with two companions: rather dingy, and too like three persons set for the camera, but powerful and deeply interesting to us, because here we see the first Medici pope, Leo X, Lorenzo de' Medici's son Giovanni, who gave Michelangelo the commission for the Medici tombs and the new Sacristy of S. Lorenzo; and in the young man on the Pope's right hand we see none other than Giulio, natural son of Giuliano de' Medici, Lorenzo's brother, who afterwards became Pope as Clement VII. It was he who laid siege to Florence when Michelangelo was called upon to fortify it; and it was during his pontificate that Henry VIII threw off the shackles of Rome and became the Defender of the Faith. Himself a bastard, Giulio became the father of the base-born Alessandro of Urbino, first Duke of Florence, who, after procuring the death of Ippolito and living a life of horrible excess, was himself murdered by his cousin Lorenzino in order to rid Florence of her worst tyrant. In his portrait Leo X has an illuminated missal and a magnifying glass, as indication of his scholarly tastes. That he was also a good liver his form and features testify.

Of this picture an interesting story is told. After the battle of Pavia, in 1525, Clement VII wishing to be friendly with the Marquis of Gonzaga, a powerful ally of the Emperor Charles V, asked him what he could do for him, and Gonzaga expressed a wish for the portrait of Leo X, then in the Medici palace. Clement complied, but wishing to retain at any rate a semblance of the original, directed that the picture should be copied, and Andrea del Sarto was chosen for that task. The copy turned out to be so close that Gonzaga never obtained the original at all.

In the next room–the Sala di Venere, and the last room in the long suite–we find another Raphael portrait, and another Pope, this time Julius II, that Pontiff whose caprice and pride together rendered null and void and unhappy so many years of Michelangelo's life, since it was for him that the great Julian tomb, never completed, was designed. A replica of this picture is in our National Gallery. Here also are a wistful and poignant John the Baptist by Dossi, No. 380; two Dürers–an Adam and an Eve, very naked and primitive, facing each other from opposite walls; and two Rubens landscapes not equal to ours at Trafalgar Square, but spacious and lively. The gem of the room is a lovely Titian, No. 92, on an easel, a golden work of supreme quietude and disguised power. The portrait is called sometimes the Duke of Norfolk, sometimes the "Young Englishman".

Returning to the first room–the Sala of the Iliad–we enter the Sala dell' Educazione di Giove, and find on the left a little gipsy portrait by Boccaccio Boccaccino (1497-1518) which has extraordinary charm: a grave, wistful, childish face in a blue handkerchief: quite a new kind of picture here. I reproduce it in this volume, but it wants its colour. For the rest, the room belongs to less-known and later men, in particular to Cristofano Allori (1577-1621), with his famous Judith, reproduced in all the picture shops of Florence. This work is no favourite of mine, but one cannot deny it power and richness. The Guido Reni opposite, in which an affected fat actress poses as Cleopatra with the asp, is not, however, even tolerable.

We next pass, after a glance perhaps at the adjoining tapestry room on the left (where the bronze Cain and Abel are), the most elegant bathroom imaginable, fit for anything rather than soap and splashes, and come to the Sala di Ulisse and some good Venetian portraits: a bearded senator in a sable robe by Paolo Veronese, No. 216, and, No. 201, Titian's fine portrait of the ill-fated Ippolito de' Medici, son of that Giuliano de' Medici, Duc de Nemours, whose tomb by Michelangelo is at S. Lorenzo. This amiable young man was brought up by Leo X until the age of twelve, when the Pope died, and the boy was sent to Florence to live at the Medici palace, with the base-born Alessandro, under the care of Cardinal Passerini, where he remained until Clarice de' Strozzi ordered both the boys to quit. In 1527 came the third expulsion of the Medici from Florence, and Ippolito wandered about until Clement VII, the second Medici Pope, was in Rome, after the sack, and, joining him there, he was, against his will, made a cardinal, and sent to Hungary: Clement's idea being to establish Alessandro (his natural son) as Duke of Florence, and squeeze Ippolito, the rightful heir, out. This, Clement succeeded in doing, and the repulsive and squalid-minded Alessandro–known as the Mule–was installed. Ippolito, in whom this proceeding caused deep grief, settled in Bologna and took to scholarship, among other tasks translating part of the Aeneid into Italian blank verse; but when Clement died and thus liberated Rome from a vile tyranny, he was with him and protected his corpse from the angry mob. That was in 1534, when Ippolito was twenty-seven. In the following year a number of exiles from Florence who could not endure Alessandro's offensive ways, or had been forced by him to fly, decided to appeal to the Emperor Charles V for assistance against such a contemptible ruler; and Ippolito headed the mission; but before he could reach the Emperor an emissary of Alessandro's succeeded in poisoning him. Such was Ippolito de' Medici, grandson of the great Lorenzo, whom Titian painted, probably when he was in Bologna, in 1533 or 1534.

This room also contains a nice little open decorative scene–like a sketch for a fresco–of the Death of Lucrezia, No. 388, attributed to the School of Botticelli, and above it a good Royal Academy Andrea del Sarto.

The next is the best of these small rooms–the Sala of Prometheus–where on Sundays most people spend their time in astonishment over the inlaid tables, but where Tuscan art also is very beautiful. The most famous picture is, I suppose, the circular Filippino Lippi, No. 343, but although the lively background is very entertaining and the Virgin most wonderfully painted, the Child is a serious blemish. The next favourite, if not the first, is the

Perugino on the easel–No. 219–one of his loveliest small pictures, with an evening glow among the Apennines such as no other painter could capture. Other fine works here are the Fra Bartolommeo, No. 256, over the door, a Holy Family, very pretty and characteristic, and his "Ecce Homo," next it; the adorable circular Botticini (as the catalogue calls it, although the photographers waver between Botticelli and Filippino Lippi), No. 347, with its myriad roses and children with their little folded hands and the Mother and Child diffusing happy sweetness, which, if only it were a little less painty, would be one of the chief magnets of the gallery.

Hereabout are many Botticelli school pictures, chief of these the curious girl, called foolishly "La Bella Simonetta," which Mr. Berenson attributes to that unknown disciple of Botticelli to whom he has given the charming name of Amico di Sandro. This study in browns, yellow, and grey always has its public. Other popular Botticelli derivatives are Nos. 348 and 357. Look also at the sly and curious woman (No. 102), near the window, by Ubertini, a new artist here; and the pretty Jacopo del Sellaio, No. 364; a finely drawn S. Sebastian by Pollaiuolo; the Holy Family by Jacopo di Boateri, No. 362, with very pleasant colouring; No. 140, the "Incognita," which people used to think was by Leonardo–for some reason difficult to understand except on the principle of making the wish father to the thought–and is now given to Bugiardini; and lastly a rich and comely example of Lombardy art, No. 299.

From this room we will enter first the Corridio delle Colonne where Cardinal Leopoldo de' Medici's miniature portraits are hung, all remarkable and some superb, but unfortunately not named, together with a few larger works, all very interesting. That Young Goldsmith, No. 207, which used to be given to Leonardo but is now Ridolfo Ghirlandaio's, is here; a Franciabigio, No. 43; a questioned Raphael, No. 44; a fine and sensitive head of one of the Gonzaga family by Mantegna, No. 375; the coarse head of Giovanni Bentivoglio by da Costa, No. 376; and a Pollaiuolo, No. 370, S. Jerome, whose fine rapt countenance is beautifully drawn.

In the Sala della Giustizia we come again to the Venetians: a noble Piombo, No. 409; the fine Aretino and Tommaso Mosti by Titian; Tintoretto's portrait of a man, No. 410; and two good Moronis. But I am not sure that Dosso Dossi's "Nymph and Satyr" on the easel is not the most remarkable achievement here. I do not, however, care greatly for it.

In the Sala di Flora we find some interesting Andreas; a beautiful portrait by Puligo, No. 184; and Giulio Romano's famous frieze of dancers. Also a fine portrait by Allori, No. 72. The end room of all is notable for a Ruysdael.

Finally there is the Sala del Poccetti, out of the Sala di Prometeo, which, together with the preceding two rooms that I have described, has lately been rearranged. Here now is the hard but masterly Holy Family of Bronzino, who has an enormous amount of work in Florence, chiefly Medicean portraits, but nowhere, I think, reaches the level of his "Allegory" in our National Gallery, or the portrait in the Taylor collection sold at Christie's in 1912. Here also are four rich Poussins; two typical Salvator Rosa landscapes and a battle piece from the same hand; and, by some strange chance, a portrait of Oliver Cromwell by Sir Peter Lely. But the stone table again wins most attention.

And here, as we leave the last of the great picture collections of Florence, I would say how interesting it is to the returned visitor to London to go quickly to the National Gallery and see how we compare with them. Florence is naturally far richer than we, but although only now and then have we the advantage, we can valuably supplement in a great many cases. And the National Gallery keeps up its quality throughout–it does not suddenly fall to pieces as the Uffizi does. Thus, I doubt if Florence with all her Andreas has so exquisite a thing from his hand as our portrait of a "Young Sculptor," so long called a portrait of the painter himself; and we have two Michelangelo paintings to the Uffizi's one. In Leonardo the Louvre is of course far richer, even without the Gioconda, but we have at Burlington House the cartoon for the Louvre's S. Anne which may pair off with the Uffizi's unfinished Madonna, and we have also at the National Gallery his finished "Virgin of the Rocks," while to Burlington House one must go too for Michelangelo's beautiful tondo. In Piero di Cosimo we are more fortunate than the Uffizi; and we have Raphaels as important as those of the Pitti. We are strong too in Perugino, Filippino Lippi, and Luca Signorelli, while when it comes to Piero della Francesca we lead absolutely. Our Verrocchio, or School of Verrocchio, is a superb thing, while our Cimabue (from S. Croce) has a quality of richness not excelled by any that I have seen elsewhere. But in Botticelli Florence wins.

The Pitti palace contains also the apartments in which the King and Queen of Italy reside when they visit Florence, which is not often. Florence became the capital of Italy in 1865, on the day of the sixth anniversary of the birth of Dante. It remained the capital until 1870, when Rome was chosen. The rooms are shown thrice a week, and are not, I think, worth the time that one must give to the perambulation. Beyond this there is nothing to say, except that they would delight children. Visitors are hurried through in small bands, and dallying is discouraged. Hence one is merely tantalized by the presence of their greatest treasure, Botticelli's "Pallas subduing the Centaur," painted to commemorate Lorenzo de' Medici's successful diplomatic mission to the King of Naples in 1480, to bring about the end of the war with Sixtus IV, the prime instigator of the Pazzi Conspiracy and the bitter enemy of Lorenzo in particular–whose only fault, as he drily expressed it, had been to "escape being murdered in the Cathedral"–and of all Tuscany in general. Botticelli, whom we have already seen as a Medicean allegorist, always ready with his glancing genius to extol and commend the virtues of that family, here makes the centaur typify war and oppression while the beautiful figure which is taming and subduing him by reason represents Pallas, or the arts of peace, here identifiable with Lorenzo by the laurel wreath and the pattern of her robe, which is composed of his private crest of diamond rings intertwined. This exquisite picture–so rich in colour and of such power and impressiveness–ought to be removed to an easel in the Pitti Gallery proper. The "Madonna della Rosa," by Botticelli or his School, is also here, and I had a moment before a very alluring Holbein. But my memory of this part of the palace is made up of gilt and tinsel and plush and candelabra, with two pieces of furniture outstanding–a blue and silver bed, and a dining table rather larger than a lawn-tennis court.

The Boboli gardens, which climb the hill from the Pitti, are also opened only on three afternoons a week. The panorama of Florence and the surrounding Apennines which one has from the Belvedere makes a visit worth while; but the gardens themselves are, from the English point of view, poor, save in extent and in the groves on the way to the stables (scuderie). Like all gardens where clipped walks are the principal feature, they want people. They were made for people to enjoy them, rather than for flowers to grow in, and at every turn there is a new and charming vista in a green frame.

It was from the Boboli hill-side before it was a garden that much of the stone of Florence was quarried. With such stones so near it is less to be wondered at that the buildings are what they are. And yet it is wonderful too–that these little inland Italian citizens should so have built their houses for all time. It proves them to have had great gifts of character. There is no such building any more.

The Grotto close to the Pitti entrance, which contains some of Michelangelo's less remarkable "Prisoners," intended for the great Julian tomb, is so "grottesque" that the statues are almost lost, and altogether it is rather an Old Rye House affair; and though Giovanni da Bologna's fountain in the midst of a lake is very fine, I doubt if the walk is quite worth it. My advice rather is to climb at once to the top, at the back of the Pitti, by way of the amphitheatre where the gentlemen and ladies used to watch court pageants, and past that ingenious fountain above it, in which Neptune's trident itself spouts water, and rest in the pretty flower garden on the very summit of the hill, among the lizards. There, seated on the wall, you may watch the peasants at work in the vineyards, and the white oxen ploughing in the olive groves, in the valley between this hill and S. Miniato. In spring the contrast between the greens of the crops and the silver grey of the olives is vivid and gladsome; in September, one may see the grapes being picked and piled into the barrels, immediately below, and hear the squdge as the wooden pestle is driven into the purple mass and the juice gushes out.

CHAPTER XXIV

ENGLISH Poets in Florence

Casa Guidi–The Brownings–Giotto's missing spire–James Russell Lowell–Lander's early life–Fra Bartolommeo before Raphael–The Tuscan gardener–The "Villa Landor" to-day–Storms on the hillside–Pastoral poetry–Italian memories in England–The final outburst–Last days in Florence–The old lion's beguilements–The famous epitaph.

On a house in the Piazza S. Felice, obliquely facing the Pitti, with windows both in the Via Maggio and Via Mazzetta, is a tablet, placed there by grateful Florence, stating that it was the home of Robert and of Elizabeth Barrett Browning and that her verse made a golden ring to link England to Italy. In other words, this is Casa Guidi.

A third member of the family, Flush the spaniel, was also with them, and they moved here in 1848, and it was here that Mrs. Browning died, in 1861. But it was not their first Florentine home, for in 1847 they had gone into rooms in the Via delle Belle Donne–the Street of Beautiful Ladies–whose name so fascinated Ruskin, near S. Maria Novella. At Casa Guidi Browning wrote, among other poems, "Christinas Eve and Easter Day," "The Statue and the Bust" of which I have said something in chapter XIX, and the "Old Pictures in Florence," that philosophic commentary on Vasari, which ends with the spirited appeal for the crowning of Giotto's Campanile with the addition of the golden spire that its builder intended–

Fine as the beak of a young beccaccia The campanile, the Duomo's fit ally, Shall soar up in gold full fifty braccia, Completing Florence, as Florence Italy.

But I suppose that the monologues "Andrea del Sarto" and "Fra Lippo Lippi" would be considered the finest fruit of Browning's Florentine sojourn, as "Casa Guidi Windows" is of Mrs. Browning's. Her great poem is indeed as passionate a plea for Italian liberty as anything by an Italian poet. Here also she wrote much if not all of "Aurora Leigh," "The Poems before Congress," and those other Italian political pieces which when her husband collected them as "Last Poems" he dedicated "to 'grateful Florence'".

In these Casa Guidi rooms the happiest days of both lives were spent, and many a time have the walls resounded to the great voice, laughing, praising or condemning, of Walter Savage Landor; while the shy Hawthorne has talked here too. Casa Guidi lodged not only the Brownings, but, at one time, Lowell, who was not, however, a very good Florentine. "As for pictures," I find him writing, in 1874, on a later visit, "I am tired to death of 'em,... and then most of them are so bad. I like best the earlier ones, that say so much in their half-unconscious prattle, and talk nature to me instead of high art." But "the older streets," he says, "have a noble mediaeval distance and reserve for me–a frown I was going to call it, not of hostility, but of haughty doubt. These grim palace fronts meet you with an aristocratic start that puts you to the proof of your credentials. There is to me something wholesome in that that makes you feel your place."

The Brownings are the two English poets who first spring to mind in connexion with Florence; but they had had very illustrious predecessors. In August and September, 1638, during the reign of Ferdinand II, John Milton was here, and again in the spring of 1639. He read Latin poems to fellow-scholars in the city and received complimentary sonnets in reply. Here he met Galileo, and from here he made the excursion to Vallombrosa which gave him some of his most famous lines. He also learned enough of the language to write love poetry to a lady in Bologna, although he is said to have offended Italians generally by his strict morality.

Skipping a hundred and eighty years we find Shelley in Florence, in 1819, and it was here that his son was born, receiving the names Percy Florence. Here he wrote, as I have said, his "Ode to the West Wind" and that grimly comic work "Peter Bell the Third".

But next the Brownings it is Walter Savage Landor of whom I always think as the greatest English Florentine. Florence became his second home when he was middle-aged and strong; and then again, when he was a very old man, shipwrecked by his impulsive and impossible temper, it became his last haven. It was Browning who found him his final resting-place–a floor of rooms not far from where we now stand, in the Via Nunziatina.

Florence is so intimately associated with Landor, and Landor was so happy in Florence, that a brief outline of his life seems to be imperative. Born in 1775, the heir to considerable estates, the boy soon developed that whirlwind headstrong impatience which was to make him as notorious as his exquisite genius has made him famous. He was sent to Rugby, but disapproving of the headmaster's judgment of his Latin verses, he produced such a lampoon upon him, also in Latin, as made removal or expulsion a necessity. At Oxford his Latin and Greek verses were still his delight, but he took also to politics, was called a mad Jacobin, and, in order to prove his sanity and show his disapproval of a person obnoxious to him, fired a gun at his shutters and was sent down for a year. He never returned. After a period of strained relations with his father and hot repudiations of all the plans for his future which were made for him–such as entering the militia, reading law, and so forth–he retired to Wales on a small allowance and wrote "Gebir" which came out in 1798, when its author was twenty-three. In 1808 Landor threw in his lot with the Spaniards against the French, saw some fighting and opened his purse for the victims of the war; but the usual personal quarrel intervened. Returning to England he bought Llanthony Abbey, stocked it with Spanish sheep, planted extensively, and was to be the squire of squires; and at the same time seeing a pretty penniless girl at a ball in Bath, he made a bet he would marry her, and won it. As a squire he became quickly involved with neighbours (an inevitable proceeding with him) and also with a Bishop concerning the restoration of the church. Lawsuits followed, and such expenses and vexations occurred that Landor decided to leave England–always a popular resource with his kind. His mother took over the estate and allowed him an income upon which he travelled from place to place for a few years, quarrelling with his wife and making it up, writing Latin verses everywhere and on everything, and coming into collision not only with individuals but with municipalities.

He settled in Florence in 1821, finding rooms in the Palazzo Medici, or, rather, Riccardi. There he remained for five years, which no doubt would have been a longer period had he not accused his landlord, the Marquis, who was then the head of the family, of seducing away his coachman. Landor wrote stating the charge; the Marquis, calling in reply, entered the room with his hat on, and Landor first knocked it off and then gave notice. It was at the Palazzo Medici that Landor was visited by Hazlitt in 1825, and here also he began the "Imaginary Conversations," his best-known work, although it is of course such brief and faultless lyrics as "Rose Aylmer" and "To Ianthe" that have given him his widest public.

On leaving the Palazzo, Landor acquired the Villa Gherardesca, on the hillside below Fiesole, and a very beautiful little estate in which the stream Affrico rises.

Crabb Robinson, the friend of so many men of genius, who was in Florence in 1880, in rooms at 1341 Via della Nuova Vigna, met Landor frequently at his villa and has left his impressions. Landor had made up his mind to live and die in Italy, but hated the Italians. He would rather, he said, follow his daughter to the grave than to her wedding with an Italian husband. Talking on art, he said he preferred John of Bologna to Michelangelo, a statement he repeated to Emerson, but afterwards, I believe, recanted. He said also to Robinson that he would not give 1000 Pounds for Raphael's "Transfiguration," but ten times that sum for Fra Bartolommeo's picture of S. Mark in the Pitti. Next to Raphael and Fra Bartolommeo he loved Perugino.

Landor soon became quite the husbandman. Writing to his sisters in 1831, he says: "I have planted 200 cypresses, 600 vines, 400 roses, 200 arbutuses, and 70 bays, besides laurustinas, etc., etc., and 60 fruit trees of the best qualities from France. I have not had a moment's illness since I resided here, nor have the children. My wife runs after colds; it would be strange if she did not take them; but she has taken none here; hers are all from Florence. I have the best water, the best air, and the best oil in the world. They speak highly of the wine too; but here I doubt. In fact, I hate wine, unless hock or claret....

"Italy is a fine climate, but Swansea better. That however is the only spot in Great Britain where we have warmth without wet. Still, Italy is the country I would live in.... In two [years] I hope to have a hundred good peaches every day at table during two months: at present I have had as many bad ones. My land is said to produce the best figs in Tuscany; I have usually six or seven bushels of them."

I have walked through Lander's little paradise–now called the Villa Landor and reached by the narrow rugged road to the right just below the village of S. Domenico. Its cypresses, planted, as I imagine, by Lander's own hand, are stately as minarets and its lawn is as green and soft as that of an Oxford college. The orchard, in April, was a mass of blossom. Thrushes sang in the evergreens and the first swallow of the year darted through the cypresses just as we reached the gates. It is truly a poet's house and garden.

In 1833 a French neighbour accused Landor of robbing him of water by stopping an underground stream, and Landor naturally challenged him to a duel. The meeting was avoided through the tact of Lander's second, the English consul at Florence, and the two men became friends. At his villa Landor wrote much of his best prose–the "Pentameron," "Pericles and Aspasia" and the "Trial of Shakespeare for Deer-stealing "–and he was in the main happy, having so much planting and harvesting to do, his children to play with, and now and then a visitor. In the main too he managed very well with the country people, but one day was amused to overhear a conversation over the hedge between two passing contadini. "All the English are mad," said one, "but as for this one...!" There was a story of Landor current in Florence in those days which depicted him, furious with a spoiled dish, throwing his cook out of the window, and then, realizing where he would fall, exclaiming in an agony, "Good God, I forgot the violets!"

Such was Landor's impossible way on occasion that he succeeded in getting himself exiled from Tuscany; but the Grand Duke was called in as pacificator, and, though the order of expulsion was not rescinded, it was not carried out.

In 1835 Landor wrote some verses to his friend Ablett, who had lent him the money to buy the villa, professing himself wholly happy–

Thou knowest how, and why, are dear to me My citron groves of Fiesole, My chirping Affrico, my beechwood nook, My Naiads, with feet only in the brook, Which runs away and giggles in their faces; Yet there they sit, nor sigh for other places–

but later in the year came a serious break. Landor's relations with Mrs. Landor, never of such a nature as to give any sense of security, had grown steadily worse as he became more explosive, and they now reached such a point that he flung out of the house one day and did not return for many years, completing the action by a poem in which he took a final (as he thought) farewell of Italy:–

I leave thee, beauteous Italy! No more From the high terraces, at even-tide, To look supine into thy depths of sky, The golden moon between the cliff and me, Or thy dark spires of fretted cypresses Bordering the channel of the milky way. Fiesole and Valdarno must be dreams, Hereafter, and my own lost Affrico Murmur to me but the poet's song.

Landor gave his son Arnold the villa, settling a sum on his wife for the other children's maintenance, and himself returned to Bath, where he added to his friends Sir William Napier (who first found a resemblance to a lion in Landor's features), John Forster, who afterwards wrote his life, and Charles Dickens, who named a child after him and touched off his merrier turbulent side most charmingly as Leonard Boythom in "Bleak House". But his most constant companion was a Pomeranian dog; in dogs indeed he found comfort all his life, right to the end.

Landor's love of his villa and estate finds expression again and again in his verse written at this time. The most charming of all these charming poems–the perfection of the light verse of a serious poet–is the letter from England to his youngest boy, speculating on his Italian pursuits. I begin at the passage describing the villa's cat:–

Does Cincirillo follow thee about, Inverting one swart foot suspensively, And wagging his dread jaw at every chirp Of bird above him on the olive-branch? Frighten him then away! 'twas he who slew Our pigeons, our white pigeons peacock-tailed, That feared not you and me–alas, nor him! I flattened his striped sides along my knee, And reasoned with him on his bloody mind, Till he looked blandly, and half-closed his eyes To ponder on my lecture in the shade. I doubt his memory much, his heart a little, And in some minor matters (may I say it?) Could wish him rather sager. But from thee God hold back wisdom yet for many years! Whether in early season or in late It always comes high-priced. For thy pure breast I have no lesson; it for me has many. Come throw it open then! What sports, what cares (Since there are none too young for these) engage Thy busy thoughts? Are you again at work, Walter and you, with those sly labourers, Geppo, Giovanni, Cecco, and Poeta, To build more solidly your broken dam Among the poplars, whence the nightingale Inquisitively watch'd you all day long? I was not of your council in the scheme, Or might have saved you silver without end,

And sighs too without number. Art thou gone Below the mulberry, where that cold pool Urged to devise a warmer, and more fit For mighty swimmers, swimming three abreast? Or art though panting in this summer noon Upon the lowest step before the hall, Drawing a slice of watermelon, long As Cupid's bow, athwart thy wetted lips (Like one who plays Pan's pipe), and letting drop The sable seeds from all their separate cells, And leaving bays profound and rocks abrupt, Redder than coral round Calypso's cave?

In 1853 Landor put forth what he thought his last book, under the title "Last Fruit off an Old Tree". Unhappily it was not his last, for in 1858 he issued yet one more, "Dry Sticks faggotted by W. S. Landor," in which was a malicious copy of verses reflecting upon a lady. He was sued for libel, lost the case with heavy damages, and once more and for the last time left England for Florence. He was now eighty-three. At first he went to the Villa Gherardesco, then the home of his son Arnold, but his outbursts were unbearable, and three times he broke away, to be three times brought back. In July, 1859, he made a fourth escape, and then escaped altogether, for Browning took the matter in hand and established him, after a period in Siena, in lodgings in the Via Nunziatina. From this time till his death in 1864 Landor may be said at last to have been at rest. He had found safe anchorage and never left it. Many friends came to see him, chief among them Browning, who was at once his adviser, his admirer and his shrewd observer. Landor, always devoted to pictures, but without much judgment, now added to his collection; Browning in one of his letters to Forster tells how he has found him "particularly delighted by the acquisition of three execrable daubs by Domenichino and Gaspar Poussin most benevolently battered by time". Another friend says that he had a habit of attributing all his doubtful pictures to Corregoio. "He cannot," Browning continues, "in the least understand that he is at all wrong, or injudicious, or unfortunate in anything.... Whatever he may profess, the thing he really loves is a pretty girl to talk nonsense with."

Of the old man in the company of fair listeners we have glimpses in the reminiscences of Mrs. Fields in the "Atlantic Monthly" in 1866. She also describes him as in a cloud of pictures. There with his Pomeranian Giallo within fondling distance, the poet, seated in his arm-chair, fired comments upon everything. Giallo's opinion was asked on all subjects, and Landor said of him that an approving wag of his tail was worth all the praise of all the "Quarterlies ". It was Giallo who led to the profound couplet–

He is foolish who supposes Dogs are ill that have hot noses.

Mrs. Fields tells how, after some classical or fashionable music had been played, Landor would come closer to the piano and ask for an old English ballad, and when "Auld Robin Gray," his favourite of all, was sung, the tears would stream down his face. "Ah, you don't know what thoughts you are recalling to the troublesome old man."

But we have Browning's word that he did not spend much time in remorse or regret, while there was the composition of the pretty little tender epigrams of this last period to amuse him and Italian politics to enchain his sympathy. His impulsive generosity led him to give his old and trusted watch to the funds for Garibaldi's Sicilian expedition; but Browning persuaded him to take it again. For Garibaldi's wounded prisoners he wrote an Italian dialogue between Savonarola and the Prior of S. Marco. The death of Mrs. Browning in 1861 sent Browning back to England, and Landor after that was less cheerful and rarely left the house. His chief solace was the novels of Anthony Trollope and G.P.R. James. In his last year he received a visit from a young English poet and enthusiast for poetry, one Algernon Charles Swinburne, who arrived in time to have a little glowing talk with the old lion and thus obtain inspiration for some fine memorial stanzas. On September 17th, 1864, Death found Landor ready–as nine years earlier he had promised it should–

To my ninth decade I have totter'd on, And no soft arm bends now my steps to steady; She who once led me where she would, is gone, So when he calls me, Death shall find me ready.

Landor was buried, as we saw, in the English cemetery within the city, whither his son Arnold was borne less than seven years later. Here is his own epitaph, one of the most perfect things in form and substance in the English language:–

I strove with none, for none was worth my strife, Nature I loved, and next to Nature, Art; I warmed both hands before the fire of life, It sinks, and I am ready to depart.

It should be cut on his tombstone.

CHAPTER XXV

THE Carmine and San Miniato

The human form divine and waxen–Galileo–Bianca Capella–A faithful Grand Duke–S. Spirito–The Carmine–Masaccio's place in art–Leonardo's summary–The S. Peter frescoes–The Pitti side–Romola–A little country walk–The ancient wall–The Piazzale Michelangelo–An evening prospect–S. Miniato–Antonio Rossellino's masterpiece–The story of S. Gualberto–A city of the dead–The reluctant departure.

The Via Maggio is now our way, but first there is a museum which I think should be visited, if only because it gave Dickens so much pleasure when he was here–the Museo di Storia Naturale, which is open three days a week only and is always free. Many visitors to Florence never even hear of it and one quickly finds that its chief frequenters are the poor. All the better for that. Here not only is the whole animal kingdom spread out before the eye in crowded cases, but the most wonderful collection of wax reproductions of the human form is to be seen. These anatomical models are so numerous and so exact that, since the human body does not change with the times, a medical student could learn everything from them in the most gentlemanly way possible. But they need a strong stomach. Mine, I confess, quailed before the end.

The hero of the Museum is Galileo, whose tomb at S. Croce we have seen: here are preserved certain of his instruments in a modern, floridly decorated Tribuna named after him. Galileo Galilei (1564-1642) belongs rather to Pisa, where he was born and where he found the Leaning Tower useful for experiments, and to Rome, where in 1611 he demonstrated his discovery of the telescope; but Florence is proud of him and it was here that he died, under circumstances tragic for an astronomer, for he had become totally blind.

The frescoes in the Tribuna celebrate other Italian scientific triumphs, and in the cases are historic telescopes, astrolabes, binoculars, and other mysteries.

The Via Maggio, which runs from Casa Guidi to the Ponte Trinita, and at noon is always full of school-girls, brings us by way of the Via Michelozzo to S. Spirito, but by continuing in it we pass a house of great interest, now No. 26, where once lived the famous Bianca Capella, that beautiful and magnetic Venetian whom some hold to have been so vile and others so much the victim of fate. Bianca Capella was born in 1543, when Francis I, Cosimo I's eldest son, afterwards to play such a part in her life, was two years of age. While he was being brought up in Florence, Bianca was gaining loveliness in her father's palace. When she was seventeen she fell in love with a young Florentine engaged in a bank in Venice, and they were secretly married. Her family were outraged by the mésalliance and the young couple had to flee to Florence, where they lived in poverty and hiding, a prize of 2000 ducats being offered by the Capella family to anyone who would kill the husband; while, by way of showing how much in earnest they were, they had his uncle thrown into prison, where he died.

One day the unhappy Bianca was sitting at her window when the young prince Francis was passing: he looked up, saw her, and was enslaved on the spot. (The portraits of Bianca do not, I must admit, lay emphasis on this story. Titian's I have not seen; but there is one by Bronzino in our National Gallery–No. 650–and many in Florence.) There was, however, something in Bianca's face to which Francis fell a victim, and he brought about a speedy meeting. At first Bianca repulsed him; but when she found that her husband was unworthy of her, she returned the Prince's affection. (I am telling her story from the pro-Bianca point of view: there are plenty of narrators on the other side.) Meanwhile, Francis's official life going on, he married that archduchess Joanna of Austria for whom the Austrian frescoes in the Palazzo Vecchio were painted; but his heart remained Bianca's and he was more at her house than in his own. At last, Bianca's husband being killed in some fray, she was free from the persecution of her family and ready to occupy the palace which Francis hastened to build for her, here, in the Via Maggio, now cut up into tenements at a few lire a week. The attachment continued unabated when Francis came to the throne, and upon the death of his archduchess in 1578 Bianca and he were almost immediately, but privately, married, she being then thirty-five; and in the next year they were publicly married in the church of S. Lorenzo with every circumstance of pomp; while later in the same year Bianca was crowned.

Francis remained her lover till his death, which was both dramatic and suspicious, husband and wife dying within a few hours of each other at the Medici villa of Poggia a Caiano in 1587. Historians have not hesitated to suggest that Francis was poisoned by his wife; but there is no proof. It is indeed quite possible that her life was more free of intrigue, ambition and falsehood, than that of any one about the court at that time; but the Florentines, encouraged by Francis's brother Ferdinand I, who succeeded him, made up their minds that she was a witch, and few things in the way of disaster happened that were not laid to her charge. Call a woman a witch and everything is possible. Ferdinand not only detested Bianca in life and deplored her fascination for his brother, but when she died he refused to allow her to be buried with the others of the family; hence the Chapel of the Princes at S. Lorenzo lacks one archduchess. Her grave is unknown.

The whole truth we shall never know; but it is as easy to think of Bianca as a harmless woman who both lost and gained through love as to picture her as sinister and scheming. At any rate we know that Francis was devoted to her with a fidelity and persistence for which Grand Dukes have not always been conspicuous.

S. Spirito is one of Brunelleschi's solidest works. Within it resembles the city of Bologna in its vistas of brown and white arches. The effect is severe and splendid; but the church is to be taken rather as architecture than a treasury of art, for although each of its eight and thirty chapels has an altar picture and several have fine pieces of sculpture–one a copy of Michelangelo's famous Pieta in Rome–there is nothing of the highest value. It was in this church that I was asked alms by one of the best-dressed men in Florence; but the Florentine beggars are not importunate: they ask, receive or are denied, and that is the end of it.

The other great church in the Pitti quarter is the Carmine, and here we are on very sacred ground in art–for it was here, as I have had occasion to say more than once in this book, that Masaccio painted those early frescoes which by their innovating boldness turned the Brancacci chapel into an Academy. For all the artists came to study and copy them: among others Michelangelo, whose nose was broken by the turbulent Torrigiano, a fellow-student, under this very roof.

Tommaso di Ser Giovanni, or Masaccio, the son of a notary, was born in 1402. His master is not known, but Tommaso Fini or Masolino, born in 1383, is often named. Vasari states that as a youth Masaccio helped Ghiberti with his first Baptistery doors; and if so, the fact is significant. But all that is really known of his early life is that he went to Rome to paint a chapel in S. Clemente. He returned, apparently on hearing that his patron Giovanni de' Medici was in power again. Another friend, Brunelleschi, having built the church of S. Spirito in 1422, Masaccio began to work there in 1423, when he was only twenty-one.

Masaccio's peculiar value in the history of painting is his early combined power of applying the laws of perspective and representing human beings "in the round". Giotto was the first and greatest innovator in painting–the father of real painting; Masaccio was the second. If from Giotto's influence a stream of vigour had flowed such as flowed from Masaccio's, there would have been nothing special to note about Masaccio at all. But the impulse which Giotto gave to art died down; some one had to reinvigorate it, and that some one was Masaccio. In his remarks on painting, Leonardo da Vinci sums up the achievements of the two. They stood out, he says, from the others of their time, by reason of their wish to go to life rather than to pictures. Giotto went to life, his followers went to pictures; and the result was a decline in art until Masaccio, who again went to life.

From the Carmine frescoes came the new painting. It is not that walls henceforth were covered more beautifully or suitably than they had been by Giotto's followers; probably less suitably very often; but that religious symbolism without much relation to actual life gave way to scenes which might credibly have occurred, where men, women and saints walked and talked much as we do, in similar surroundings, with backgrounds of cities that could be lived in and windows that could open. It was this revolution that Masaccio performed. No doubt if he had not, another would, for it had to come: the new demand was that religion should be reconciled with life.

It is generally supposed that Masaccio had Masolino as his ally in this wonderful series; and a vast amount of ink has been spilt over Masolino's contributions. Indeed the literature of expert art criticism on Florentine pictures alone is of alarming bulk and astonishing in its affirmations and denials. The untutored visitor in the presence of so much scientific variance will be wise to enact the part of the lawyer in the old caricature of the litigants and the cow, who, while they pull, one at the head and the other at the tail, fills his bucket with milk. In other words, the plain duty of the ordinary person is to enjoy the picture.

Without any special knowledge of art one can, by remembering the early date of these frescoes, realize what excitement they must have caused in the studios and how tongues must have clacked in the Old Market. We have but to send our thoughts to the Spanish chapel at S. Maria Novella to realize the technical advance. Masaccio, we see, was peopling a visible world; the Spanish chapel painters were merely allegorizing, as agents of holiness. The Ghirlandaio choir in the same church would yield a similar comparison; but what we have to remember is that Ghirlandaio painted these frescoes in 1490, sixty-two years after Masaccio's death, and Masaccio showed him how.

It is a pity that the light is so poor and that the frescoes have not worn better; but their force and dramatic vigour remain beyond doubt. The upper scene on the left of the altar is very powerful: the Roman tax collector has asked Christ for a tribute and Christ bids Peter find the money in the mouth of a fish. Figures, architecture, landscape, all are in right relation; and the drama is moving, without restlessness. This and the S. Peter preaching and distributing alms are perhaps the best, but the most popular undoubtedly is that below it, finished many years after by Filippino Lippi (although there are experts to question this and even substitute his amorous father), in which S. Peter, challenged by Simon Magus, resuscitates a dead boy, just as S. Zenobius used to do in the streets of this city. Certain more modern touches, such as the exquisite Filippino would naturally have thought of, may be seen here: the little girl behind the boy, for instance, who recalls the children in that fresco by the same hand at S. Maria Novella in which S. John resuscitates Drusiana. In this Carmine fresco are many portraits of Filippino's contemporaries, including Botticelli, just as in the scene of the consecration of the Carmine which Masaccio painted in the cloisters, but which has almost perished, he introduced Brancacci, his employer, Brunelleschi, Donatello, some of whose innovating work in stone he was doing in paint, Giovanni de' Medici and Masolino. The scanty remains of this fresco tell us that it must have been fine indeed.

Masaccio died at the early age of twenty-six, having suddenly disappeared from Florence, leaving certain work unfinished. A strange portentous meteor in art.

The Pitti side of the river is less interesting than the other, but it has some very fascinating old and narrow streets, although they are less comfortable for foreigners to wander in than those, for example, about the Borgo SS. Apostoli. They are far dirtier.

From the Pitti end of the Ponte Vecchio one can obtain a most charming walk. Turn to the left as you leave the bridge, under the arch made by Cosimo's passage, and you are in the Via de' Bardi, the backs of whose houses on the river-side are so beautiful from the Uffizi's central arches, as Mr. Morley's picture shows. At the end of the street is an archway under a large house. Go through this, and you are at the foot of a steep, stone hill. It is really steep, but never mind. Take it easily, and rest half-way where the houses on the left break and give a wonderful view of the city. Still climbing, you come to the best gate of all that is left–a true gate in being an inlet into a fortified city–that of S. Giorgio, high on the Boboli hill by the fort. The S. Giorgio gate has a S. George killing a dragon, in stone, on its outside, and the saint painted within, Donatello's conception of him being followed by the artist. Parsing through, you are in the country. The fort and gardens are on one side and villas on the other; and a great hill-side is in front, covered with crops. Do not go on, but turn sharp to the left and follow the splendid city wall, behind which for a long way is the garden of the Villa Karolath, one of the choicest spots in Florence, occasionally tossing its branches over the top. This wall is immense all the way down to the Porta S. Miniato, and two of the old towers are still standing in their places upon it. Botticini's National Gallery picture tells exactly how they looked in their heyday. Ivy hangs over, grass and flowers spring from the ancient stones, and lizards run about. Underneath are olive-trees.

It was, by the way, in the Via de' Bardi that George Eliot's Romola lived, for she was of the Bardi family. The story, it may be remembered, begins on the morning of Lorenzo the Magnificent's death, and ends after the execution of Savonarola. It is not an inspired romance, and is remarkable almost equally for its psychological omissions and the convenience of its coincidences, but it is an excellent preparation for a first visit in youth to S. Marco and the Palazzo Vecchio, while the presence in its somewhat naive pages of certain Florentine characters makes it agreeable to those who know something of the city and its history. The painter Piero di Cosimo, for example, is here, straight from Vasari; so also are Cronaca, the architect, Savonarola, Capparo, the ironsmith, and even Machiavelli; while Bernardo del Nero, the gonfalonier, whose death sentence Savonarola refused to revise, was Romola's godfather.

The Via Guicciardini, which runs from the foot of the Via de' Bardi to the Pitti, is one of the narrowest and busiest Florentine streets, with an undue proportion of fruit shops overflowing to the pavement to give it gay colouring. At No. 24 is a stable with pillars and arches that would hold up a pyramid. But this is no better than most of the old stables of Florence, which are all solid vaulted caverns of immense size and strength.

From the Porta Romana one may do many things–take the tram, for example, for the Certosa of the Val d'Ema, which is only some twenty minutes distant, or make a longer journey to Impruneta, where the della Robbias are. But just now let us walk or ride up the long winding Viale Macchiavelli, which curves among the villas behind the Boboli Gardens, to the Piazzale Michelangelo and S. Miniato.

The Piazzale Michelangelo is one of the few modern tributes of Florence to her illustrious makers. The Dante memorial opposite S. Croce is another, together with the preservation of certain buildings with Dante associations in the heart of the city; but, as I have said more than once, there is no piazza in Florence, and only one new street, named after a Medici. From the Piazzale Michelangelo you not only have a fine panoramic view of the city of this great man–in its principal features not so vastly different from the Florence of his day, although of course larger and with certain modern additions, such as factory chimneys, railway lines, and so forth–but you can see the remains of the fortifications which he constructed in 1529, and which kept the Imperial troops at bay for nearly a year. Just across the river rises S. Croce, where the great man is buried, and beyond, over the red roofs, the dome of the Medici chapel at S. Lorenzo shows us the position of the Biblioteca Laurenziana and the New Sacristy, both built by him. Immediately below us is the church of S. Niccolo, where he is said to have hidden in 1529, when there was a hue and cry for him. In the middle of this spacious plateau is a bronze reproduction of his David, and it is good to see it, from the cafe behind it, rising head and shoulders above the highest Apennines.

S. Miniato, the church on the hill-top above the Piazzale Michelangelo, deserves many visits. One may not be too greatly attached to marble façades, but this little temple defeats all prejudices by its radiance and perfection, and to its extraordinary charm its situation adds. It crowns the hill, and in the late afternoon–the ideal time to visit it–is full in the eye of the sun, bathed in whose light the green and white façade, with miracles of delicate intarsia, is balm to the eyes instead of being, as marble so often is, dazzling and cold.

On the way up we pass the fine church of S. Salvatore, which Cronaca of the Palazzo Vecchio and Palazzo Strozzi built and Michelangelo admired, and which is now secularized, and pass through the gateway of Michelangelo's upper fortifications. S. Miniato is one of the oldest churches of Florence, some of it eleventh century. It has its name from Minias, a Roman soldier who suffered martyrdom at Florence under Decius. Within, one does not feel quite to be in a Christian church, the effect partly of the unusual colouring, all grey, green, and gold and soft light tints as of birds' bosoms; partly of the ceiling, which has the bright hues of a Russian toy; partly of the forest of great gay columns; partly of the lovely and so richly decorated marble screen; and partly of the absence of a transept. The prevailing feeling indeed is gentle gaiety; and in the crypt this is intensified, for it is just a joyful assemblage of dancing arches.

The church as a whole is beautiful and memorable enough; but its details are wonderful too, from the niello pavement, and the translucent marble windows of the apse, to the famous tomb of Cardinal Jacopo of Portugal, and the Luca della Robbia reliefs of the Virtues. This tomb is by Antonio Rossellino. It is not quite of the rank of Mino's in the Badia; but it is a noble and beautiful thing marked in every inch of it by modest and exquisite thought. Vasari says of Antonio that he "practised his art with such grace that he was valued as something more than a man by those who knew him, who well-nigh adored him as a saint". Facing it is a delightful Annunciation by Alessio Baldovinetti, in which the angel declares the news from a far greater distance than we are accustomed to; and the ceiling is made an abode of gladness by the blue and white figures (designed by Luca della Robbia) of Prudence and Chastity, Moderation and Fortitude, for all of which qualities, it seems, the Cardinal was famous. In short, one cannot be too glad that, since he had to die, death's dart struck down this Portuguese prelate while he was in Rossellino's and Luca's city.

No longer is preserved here the miraculous crucifix which, standing in a little chapel in the wood on this spot, bestowed blessing and pardon–by bending towards him–upon S. Giovanni Gualberto, the founder of the Vallombrosan order. The crucifix is now in S. Trinita. The saint was born in 985 of noble stock and assumed naturally the splendour and arrogance of his kind. His brother Hugo being murdered in some affray, Giovanni took upon himself the duty of avenging the crime. One Good Friday he chanced to meet, near this place, the assassin, in so narrow a passage as to preclude any chance of escape; and he was about to kill him when the man fell on his knees and implored mercy by the passion of Christ Who suffered on that very day, adding that Christ had prayed on the cross for His own murderers. Giovanni was so much impressed that he not only forgave the man but offered him his friendship. Entering then the chapel to pray and ask forgiveness of all his sins, he was amazed to see the crucifix bend down as though acquiescing and blessing, and this special mark of favour so wrought upon him that he became a monk, himself shaving his head for that purpose and defying his father's rage, and subsequently founded the Vallombrosan order. He died in 1073.

I have said something of the S. Croce habit and the S. Maria Novella habit; but I think that when all is said the S. Miniato habit is the most important to acquire. There is nothing else like it; and the sense of height is so invigorating too. At all times of the year it is beautiful; but perhaps best in early spring, when the highest mountains still have snow upon them and the neighbouring slopes are covered with tender green and white fruit blossom, and here the violet wistaria blooms and there the sombre crimson of the Judas-tree.

Behind and beside the church is a crowded city of the Florentine dead, reproducing to some extent the city of the Florentine living, in its closely packed habitations–the detached palaces for the rich and the great congeries of cells for the poor–more of which are being built all the time. There is a certain melancholy interest in wandering through these silent streets, peering through the windows and recognizing over the vaults names famous in Florence. One learns quickly how bad modern mortuary architecture and sculpture can be, but I noticed one monument with some sincerity and unaffected grace: that to a charitable Marchesa, a friend of the poor, at the foot of whose pedestal are a girl and baby done simply and well.

Better perhaps to remain on the highest point and look at the city beneath. One should try to be there before sunset and watch the Apennines turning to a deeper and deeper indigo and the city growing dimmer and dimmer in the dusk. Florence is beautiful from every point of vantage, but from none more beautiful than from this eminence. As one reluctantly leaves the church and passes again through Michelangelo's fortification gateway to descend, one has, framed in its portal, a final lovely Apennine scene.

Historical Chart of Florence and Europe, 1296-1564

Artists' Dates.

1300 (c.) Taddeo Gaddi born (d. 1366) 1302 (c.) Cimabue died (b. c. 1240) 1308 (c.) Andrea Orcagna born (d. 1368) 1310 Arnolfo di Cambio died (b. 1232 ?) 1333 Spinello Aretino born (d. 1410) 1336 Giotto died (b. 1276 ?) 1344 Simone Martini died (b. 1283) 1348 Andrea Pisano died (b. 1270) 1356 Lippo Memmi died 1366 Taddeo Gaddi died (b. c. 1300) 1368 Andrea Orcagna died 1370 (c.) Lorenzo Monaco born (d. 1425) Gentile da Fabriano born (d.

1450) 1371 Jacopo della Quercia born (d. 1438) 1377 Filippo Brunelleschi born (d. 1446) 1378 Lorenzo Ghiberti born (d. 1455) 1386 (?) Donatello born (d. 1466) 1387 Fra Angelico born (d. 1455) 1391 Michelozzo born (d. 1472) 1396 (?) Andrea del Castagno born (d. 1457) 1397 Paolo Uccello born (d. 1475) 1399 or 1400 Luca della Robbia born (d. 1482) 1401 or 1402 Masaccio born (d. 1428?) 1405 Leon Battista Alberti born (d. 1472) 1406 Lippo Lippi born (d. 1469) 1409 Bernardo Rossellino born (d. 1464) 1410 Spinello Aretino died 1415 Piero della Francesca born (d. 1492) 1420 Benozzo Gozzoli born (d. 1498) 1425 Il Monaco died Alessio Baldovinetti born (d. 1499) 1427 Antonio Rossellino born (d. 1478) 1428 (?) Masaccio died 1428 Desiderio da Settignano born (d. 1464) 1429 (?) Giovanni Bellini born (d. 1516) Antonio Pollaiuolo born (d. 1498) 1430 Cosimo Tura died 1431 Andrea Mantegna born (d. 1506) 1432 (?) Mina da Fiesole born (d. 1484) 1435 Andrea Verrocchio born (d. 1488) Andrea della Robbia born (d. 1525) 1438 Melozzo da Forli born (d. 1494) 1439 Cosimo Rosselli born (d. 1507) 1441 Luca Signorelli born (d. 1523) 1442 Benedetto da Maiano born (d. 1497) 1444 Sandro Botticelli born (d. 1510) 1446 Brunelleschi died Perugino born (d. 1523 or 24) Francesco Botticini born (d. 1498) 1449 Domenico Ghirlandaio born (d. 1494) 1450 Gentile da Fabriano died 1452 Leonardi da Vinci born (d. 1519) 1455 Ghiberti died Fra Angelico died 1456 Lorenzo di Credi born (d. 1537) 1457 Cronaca born (d. 1508 or 9) Filippino Lippi born (d. 1504) Andrea del Castagno died 1462 Piero di Cosimo born (d. 1521) 1463 or 4 Desiderio da Settignano died 1464 Bernardo Rossellino died 1466 Donatello died 1469 Giovanni della Robbia born (d. 1529) Lippo Lippi died 1472 Michelozzo died Alberti died 1474 Benedetto da Rovezzano born (d. 1556) Rustici born (d. 1554) Mariotto Albertinelli born (d. 1515) 1475 Fra Bartolommeo born (d. 1517) Michelangelo Buonarroti born (d. 1564) 1477 Titian born (d. 1576) Giorgione born (d. 1510) 1478 Antonio Rossellino died 1482 Francia Bigio born (d. 1523) Guicciardini born (d. 1540) 1483 Raphael born (d. 1520) Ridolfo Ghirlandaio born (d. 1561) 1484 Mino da Fiesole died 1485 Sebastiano del Piombo born (d. 1547) 1486 Jacopo Sansovino born (d. 1570) 1486 or 7 Andrea del Sarto born (d. 1531) 1488 Verrocchio died Baccio Bandinelli born

(d. 1560) 1492 Piero della Francesco died 1494 Jacopo da Pontormo born (d. 1556) Correggio born (d. 1534) Domenico Ghirlandaio died Melozzo da Forli died 1497 Benedetto da Maiano died Benozzo Gozzoli died 1498 Antonio Pollaiuolo died Francesco Botticini died 1499 Alessio Baldovinetti died 1500 Benvenuto Cellini born (d. 1572) 1502 Angelo Bronzino born (d. 1572) 1504 Filippino Lippi died 1506 Mantegna died 1507 Cosimo Rosselli died 1508 Cronaca died 1510 Botticelli died Giorgione died 1511 Vasari born (d. 1574) 1515 Albertinelli died 1516 Giovanni Bellini died 1517 Fra Bartolommeo died 1518 Tintoretto born (d. 1594) 1519 Leonardo da Vinci died 1520 Raphael died 1521 Piero di Cosimo died 1523 Signorelli died Perugino died 1524 Giovanni da Bologna born (d. 1608) 1525 Andrea della Robbia died Francia Bigio died 1528 Paolo Veronese born (d. 1588) Federigo Baroccio born (d. 1612) 1529 Giovanni della Robbia died 1531 Andrea del Sarto died 1534 Correggio died 1537 Credi died 1547 Sebastiano del Piombo died 1554 Rustici died 1556 Pontormo died Benedetto da Rovezzano died 1560 Baccio Bandinelli died 1561 Ridolfo Ghirlandaio died 1564 Michael Angelo died

Some Important Florentine Dates

1296 Foundations of the Duomo consecrated 1298 Palazzo Vecchio commenced by Arnolfo di Cambio 1300 Beginning of the feuds of the Bianchi and Xeri Guido Cavalcanti died 1302 Dante exiled, Jan. 27 1304 Petrarch born (d. 1374) 1308 Death of Corso Donati 1312 Siege of Florence by Henry VII 1313 Boccaccio born (d. 1375) 1321 Dante died Sept. 14 (b. 1265) 1333 Destructive floods 1334 Foundations of the Campanile laid 1337 Or San Michele begun 1339 Andrea Pisano's gates finished 1348 Black Death of the Decameron Giovanni Villani died (b. 1275 c.) 1360 Giovanni de' Medici (di Bicci) born 1365 (c) Ponte Vecchio rebuilt by Taddeo Gaddi 1374 Petrarch died 1375 Boccaccio died 1376 Loggia de' Lanzi commenced 1378 Salvestro de' Medici elected Gonfaloniere 1389 Cosimo de' Medici (Pater Patrise) born 1390 War with Milan 1394 Sir John Hawkwood died 1399 Competition for Baptistery Gates 1416 Piero de' Medici (il Gottoso) born 1421 Purchase of Leghorn by Florence Giovanni de' Medici elected Gonfaloniere Spedale degli Innocenti commenced 1424 Ghiberti's first gate set up 1429 Giovanni de' Medici died 1432 Niccolo da Uzzano died 1433 Marsilio Ficino born Cosimo de' Medici banished, Oct. 3 1434 Cosimo returned to power, Sept. 29 Banishment of Albizzi and Strozzi 1435 Francesco Sforza visited Florence 1436 Brunelleschi's dome completed The Duomo consecrated 1439 Council of Florence Gemisthos Plethon in Florence 1440 Cosimo occupied the Medici Palace 1449 Lorenzo de' Medici (the Magnificent born) 1452 Ghiberti's second gates set up Savonarola born 1454 Politian born 1463 Pico della Mirandola born 1464 Cosimo de' Medici died and was succeeded by Piero 1466 Luca Pitti's Conspiracy 1469 Lorenzo's Tournament, Feb. Lorenzo's Marriage to Clarice Orsini, June Death of Piero, Dec. Niccolò Machiavelli born 1471 Piero de' Medici, son of Lorenzo, born Visit of Galeazzo Sforza to Florence Cennini's Press established in Florence 1474 Ariosto born 1475 Giuliano's Tournament 1478 Pazzi Conspiracy Giuliano murdered 1479 Lorenzo's Mission to Naples 1492 Lorenzo the Magnificent died Piero succeeded 1494 Charles VIII invaded Italy Piero banished Charles VIII in Florence. Sack of Medici Palace Florence governed by General Council Savonarola in power Politian died Pico della Mirandola died 1497 Francesco Valori elected Gonfaloniere Piero attempted to return to Florence 1498 Savonarola burnt 1499 Marsilio Ficino died Amerigo Vespucci reached America 1503 Death of Piero di Medici 1512 Cardinal Giovanni and Giuliano, Duke of Nemours, reinstated in Florence Great Council abolished 1519 Cardinal Giulio de' Medici in power Catherine de' Medici born 1524 Ippolito and Alessandro de' Medici in power 1526 Death of Giovanni delle Bande Nere 1527 Ippolito and Alessandro left Florence 1528 Machiavelli died 1529-30 Siege of Florence 1530 Capitulation of Florence 1531 Alessandro de' Medici declared Head of Republic 1537 Cosimo de' Medici made Ruler of Florence Battle of Montemurlo Lorenzino assassinated in Venice 1539 Cosimo married Eleanor di Toledo and moved to Palazzo Vecchio 1553 Cosimo occupied the Pitti Palace 1564 Galileo Galilei born

Popes.

Boniface VIII 1303 Benedict XI 1305 Clement V 1316 John XXII 1334 Benedict XII 1337 Boniface VIII 1342 Clement VI 1352 Innocent VI 1362 Urban V 1370 Gregory XI 1378 Urban VI 1389 Boniface IX 1404 Innocent VII 1406 Gregory XII 1409 Alex. V 1410 John XXIII 1417 Martin V 1431 Eugenius IV 1447 Nicolas V 1455 Calixtus III 1458 Pius II 1464 Paul II 1471 Sixtus IV 1484 Innocent VIII 1492 Alex. VI 1503 Pius III Julius II 1513 Leo X 1522 Hadrian VI 1523 Clement VII 1534 Paul III 1550 Julius III 1555 Marcellus II Paul IV 1559 Pius IV

French Kings.

Philip IV 1314 Louis X 1316 John I Philip V 1322 Charles IV 1328 Philip VI Philip 1350 John II 1364 Charles V 1380 Charles VI 1422 Charles VII 1461 Louis XI 1483 Charles VIII 1498 Louis XII 1515 Francis I 1547 Henry II 1559 Francis II 1560 Charles IX

English Kings.

Edward I 1307 Edward II 1327 Edward III 1377 Richard II 1422 Charles VII 1461 Edward IV 1483 Edward V Richard III 1485 Henry VII 1509 Henry VIII 1547 Edward VI 1553 Mary 1558 Elizabeth

Milan.

1310 Matteo Visconti 1322 Galeazzo Visconti 1328 1329 Azzo Visconti 1339 Luchino and Giovanni Visconti 1349 Giovanni Visconti 1354 Matteó Bernabò Galeazzo 1378 Gian Galeazzo Visconti 1402 Gian Maria Visconti 1412 Filippo Maria Visconti 1447...1450 Francesco Sforza 1466 Galeazzo Sforza 1476 Gian Galeazzo Sforza (Ludovico Sforza Regent) 1495 Ludovico Sforza 1499 Ludovico exiled

Some Important General Dates

1298 Battle of Falkirk 1306 Coronation of Bruce 1314 Battle of Bannockburn 1324 (?) John Wyclif born 1337 Froissart born (d. 1410?) 1339 Beginning of the Hundred Years' War 1346 Battle of Crécy 1347 Rienzi made Tribune of Rome Edward III took Calais 1348-9 Black Death in England 1348 S. Catherine of

Siena born 1356 Battle of Poictiers 1362 First draft of Piers Plowman 1379 Thomas à Kempis born 1381 Wat Tyler's Rebellion 1400 Geoffrey Chaucer died 1414 Council of Constance 1428 Siege of Orléans 1431 Joan of Arc burnt 1435 (c.) Hans Meinling born 1450 John Gutenburg printed at Mainz Jack Cade's Insurrection 1453 Fall of Constantinople 1455 Beginning of the Wars of the Roses 1467 Erasmus born (d. 1528) 1470 (c.) Mabuse born (d. 1555) 1471 Albert Dürer born (d. 1528) Caxton's Press established in Westminster 1476 Chevalier Bayard born 1482 Hugo van der Goes died 1483 Rabelais born (d. 1553) Martin Luther born Murder of the Princes in the Tower 1491 Ignatius Loyola born 1492 America discovered by Christopher Columbus 1494 Lucas van Leyden born (d. 1533) 1505 John Knox born (d. 1582) 1509 Calvin born 1516 More's Utopia published 1519 First Voyage round the world (Ferd. Magellan) 1519-21 Conquest of Mexico 1520 Field of the Cloth of Gold 1527 Brantôme born (d. 1614) 1528 Albert Dürer died 1531-2 Conquest of Peru 1533 Montaigne born (d. 1592) 1535 Henry VIII became Supreme Head of the Church 1537 Sack of Rome 1544 Torquato Tasso born 1553 Edmund Spenser born 1554 Execution of Lady Jane Grey Sir Philip Sidney born 1555-6 Ridley, Latimer, Cranmer burnt 1558 Calais recaptured by the French 1564 Shakespeare born

NOTES

[1] One of Brunelleschi's devices to bring before the authorities an idea of the dome he projected, was of standing an egg on end, as Columbus is famed for doing, fully twenty years before Columbus was born.

[2] It was Charles V who said of Giotto's Campanile that it ought to be kept in a glass case.

[3] Hence its new name: Loggia de' Lanzi.

[4] In the Victoria and Albert Museum at South Kensington are casts of the two Medici on the tombs and also the Madonna and Child. They are in the great gallery of the casts, together with the great David, two of the Julian tomb prisoners, the Bargello tondo and the Brutus.

[5] Cacus, the son of Vulcan and Medusa, was a famous robber who breathed fire and smoke and laid waste Italy. He made the mistake, however, of robbing Hercules of some cows, and for this Hercules strangled him.

[6] "Thick as leaves in Vallombrosa" has come to be the form of words as most people quote them. But Milton wrote ("Paradise Lost," Book I. 300-304):–

"He called His legions, angel-forms, who lay entranced Thick as autumnal leaves that strew the brooks In Vallombrosa where the Etrurian shades, High over-arched, embower."

Wordsworth, by the way, when he visited Vallombrosa with Crabb Robinson in 1837, wrote an inferior poem there, in a rather common metre, in honour of Milton's association with it.

[7] 27 April, 1859, the day that the war with Austria was proclaimed.

[8] In "A Dictionary of Saintly Women".

[9] The position of easel pictures in the Florentine galleries often changes.

www.ingramcontent.com/pod-product-compliance
Lightning Source LLC
LaVergne TN
LVHW050801061126
851857LV00012B/639

* 9 7 8 3 9 8 0 8 6 9 0 6 5 *